Katrina's Imprint

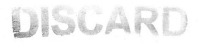

Rutgers Studies in Race and Ethnicity

Controversies in race and ethnicity cannot be fully understood through a single analytical lens or disciplinary approach. Such issues require sustained, collaborative analysis—drawing on insights from law to history, from sociology to literature, from labor studies to anthropology, from political science to health-related scholarship, and from biology to cultural studies. Focusing primarily on edited volumes, the series aims to bring multiple theories, methods, and approaches to bear on how racial and ethnic politics, identity, culture, structures, and social relations function in the modern world. Through innovative critical commentary and sustained policy engagement, this series encourages scholarship aimed at expanding and deepening the study of these issues in the United States and around the globe. Organized by the Rutgers Center for Race and Ethnicity, the series is an outgrowth of the breadth, depth, and strength of the field at the University and is committed to new collaborative scholarship that bridges boundaries. Readers will find a deep and expansive understanding of the intricate and often unrecognized ways in which race and ethnicity shapes and is shaped by modern societies.

Series Editors: Keith Wailoo, Karen M. O'Neill, Mia Bay, and Lisa Miller

Keith Wailoo, Karen M. O'Neill, Jeffrey Dowd, and Roland Anglin, eds., *Katrina's Imprint: Race and Vulnerability in America*

Katrina's Imprint

Race and Vulnerability in America

EDITED BY
KEITH WAILOO
KAREN M. O'NEILL
JEFFREY DOWD
ROLAND ANGLIN

RUTGERS UNIVERSITY PRESS

NEW BRUNSWICK, NEW JERSEY, AND LONDON

LIBRARY OF CONGRESS CATALOGING-IN-PUBLICATION DATA

Katrina's imprint : race and vulnerability in America / edited by
Keith Wailoo . . . [et al.].
   p. cm. — (Rutgers studies in race and ethnicity)
   Includes bibliographical references and index.
   ISBN 978–0–8135–4773–2 (hbk. : alk. paper) — ISBN 978–0–8135–4774–9
(pbk. : alk. paper)
   1. Hurricane Katrina, 2005—Social aspects.   2. Disaster relief—Social
aspects—Louisiana—New Orleans.   3. Disaster relief—Social aspects—Gulf States.
4. United States—Social conditions—21st century.   I. Wailoo, Keith.
   HV636 2005 .N4 K38 2010
   976'.044—dc22   2009038466

A British Cataloging-in-Publication record for this book is available
from the British Library.

Visit our Web site: http://rutgerspress.rutgers.edu

Manufactured in the United States of America

CONTENTS

ACKNOWLEDGMENTS

This project—an analysis of the enduring significance of Katrina in American society—originated in a May 2006 conference organized by the then newly created Center for Race and Ethnicity at Rutgers, The State University of New Jersey. Participants in that conference included the authors in this volume as well as many others. The conference presentations of Donna Murch, Dorothy Sue Cobble, Alison Isenberg, Minkah Makalani, James K. Mitchell, and Nancy Sinkoff helped demonstrate the benefits of the multidisciplinary approach of this volume. Among the authors in this volume, we especially thank Richard Mizelle, who, as a postdoctoral fellow at the Center for Race and Ethnicity, taught a multidisciplinary course on Katrina that involved several of the authors in this volume and provided an exciting forum to continue the investigation that had begun in May 2006. As well, we thank Maureen Dekaser and Mia Kissil for assistance with organizing the conferences and the course that gave rise to this volume. Mia Bay also warrants special thanks for her essential part in organizing this project and planning this book. Several graduate students assisted with research. We would like to recognize and thank Daniel Wherley, who carried out a great deal of research for several of the authors, as well as Rebecca Scales, Marc Matera, and Joseph Gabriel. Several other graduate students played a major role in editing, commenting, and assisting with revisions. In particular, we thank Shakti Jaising for her extraordinarily insightful contribution as copy editor, Anantha Sudhakar, Fatimah Williams-Castro, Isra Ali, Dana Brown, Bridget Gurtler, Dora Vargha, Melissa Stein, and Nadia Brown. Jeffrey Dowd began as a graduate assistant and copy editor, and as his involvement with the essays and the volume expanded, he became a coeditor and coauthor. We are especially indebted to Jeff for his work in this regard. We would also like to thank Leslie Mitchner, editor-in-chief at Rutgers University Press, for her insights and suggestions on particular essays as well as on the overall structure of the book. Finally, this project would not have been possible without strong support for the Center for Race and Ethnicity by Rutgers President Richard L. McCormick and Executive Vice President for Academic Affairs Philip Furmanski.

Katrina's Imprint

Introduction

Katrina's Imprint

KEITH WAILOO

KAREN M. O'NEILL

JEFFREY DOWD

The mention of Hurricane Katrina conjures up more than just a violent storm that unleashed nature's destructive force on an American city. Hurricane Katrina is now also recalled as a political event that issued a black mark on a presidency, an epic media story that produced collective trauma far beyond those physically affected, a breakdown of order that shredded the American social fabric (as demonstrated by the divergent reactions of black and white Americans), and an economic calamity that has produced one of the most dramatic urban transformations in modern times. Finally, Katrina is a shameful episode, unparalleled in American history; nevertheless (as authors in this volume insist), it cannot be isolated from earlier calamities nor from the mundane realities of American life and history.

The problems that Katrina highlighted are not new; rather, the storm was merely the latest manifestation of a set of patterns whereby poverty and other varieties of inequality come suddenly—and fleetingly—into view. As Michael Harrington wrote nearly a half-century ago, "There are mighty historical and economic forces that keep the poor down; and there are human beings who help out in this grim business, many of them unwittingly. There are sociological and political reasons why poverty is not seen; and there are misconceptions and prejudices that literally blind the eyes. The latter must be understood if anyone is to make the necessary act of intellect and will so that the poor can be noticed."[1] Katrina was one of those moments when deeply structured inequalities (in housing, in environmental exposures, in access to health care and transportation, and in media coverage) and suffering poor people themselves came briefly and tragically into view. Unfortunately, as David Troutt argues in this volume, "what Katrina threatened to reveal about hardship, community, and self-sufficiency in about five raw and agonizing days of news coverage has assumed [years later] its invisible form again." Yet, even though the poor have once again faded from view in subsequent years, Katrina (the event and the issues it symbolizes) will continue to resonate in the American psyche for decades to come.

The contributors to this book came together just months after the storm struck to reflect on the then-recent events and to discuss our shared experiences of the storm through the lenses of our specialties—from history to political science, from law to psychology. Like many Americans, we were overwhelmed by the immensity and complexity of the disaster. However, many of us knew from our own research that New Orleans and other parts of the Gulf Coast had already been experiencing a slow-moving, multigenerational disaster, which has visited poverty, poor health, and environmental vulnerability on so many. We set about, in a systematic and sustained way, to learn from Katrina. In the course of this sustained reflection, we came to understand just how much Katrina said about our society. We also realized that our disparate expertise and understandings (of nonprofit organizations, of transportation, of health care, and of labor markets) were linked by common questions about the social and political origins of vulnerability.

The essays in this volume enhance our understanding of Katrina's imprint—situating the origins of Katrina in the deep American past but also looking forward and away from the Mississippi Gulf region to the larger social forces that give meaning to such troubling events. In these essays we learn, for example, that the logic of vulnerability is a vast web of interconnecting vulnerabilities—spanning environmental injustice and the risk embedded in our nation's transportation and health-care systems—and that these vulnerabilities are accentuated by the structure of our federal system of governance. As Roland Anglin notes, "The system is not set up to manage long-term ecological and social challenges." We learn also that the trauma of Katrina was multifaceted—from the shock of seeing dead bodies in the media, to experiencing forced displacement and loss of home, to the "vicarious racism" examined by Nancy Boyd-Franklin. Finally, we learn that these experiences were traumatic precisely because they evoked, built on, and resonated with a troubling past for African Americans in the Gulf area and beyond. The lack of a feasible evacuation plan for poor residents of New Orleans, described in detail by Mia Bay, reminds many of the past restrictions on African Americans' travel in the South. The visible evidence of abandoned houses, which Evie Shockley presents as a lasting symbol of the disaster, recalls many historical moments when larger social forces displaced blacks from their homes. The diaspora of former residents of the Gulf Coast, analyzed by Niki Dickerson, parallels the African diaspora of slavery. Yet, while Katrina evoked uncomfortable truths about race for all Americans, it also called on Americans to be resilient and to focus on healing and recovery.

But most important, these essays reveal that because Katrina was the product of flawed structural and cultural systems, any notion of recovery and rebuilding will be fraught. For, after all, what does it mean to "rebuild" a city that was both an icon of African American life and an embodiment of structured vulnerabilities? This tension over how to think about Katrina, what lessons it teaches, and how to build anew runs throughout the essays in this volume. The tension becomes particularly evident in the continuing invocation of Katrina in the media, politics, and popular culture. In media coverage of more recent floods, fires, and other disasters, we find that Katrina's meaning is constantly changing. To invoke Katrina, therefore, is to continue a debate that started with the storm: about the role of government and the private sector, about the role of race in structured vulnerability, and about the problem of recovery, relocation, and the challenge of starting over.

As many of the essays in this volume highlight, Katrina allows us to see that the cherished myths of Americans—self-sufficiency, free enterprise, individual initiative, starting over—are themselves heavily subsidized by government. That is, beneath these myths is the reality of government policies (on land use, transportation, health care, and housing) that have created the economic possibilities for developers and middle-class citizens to freely travel and build as they have. Mia Bay's essay (showing how heavy subsidies for highways and for evacuation by private automobile enabled some to flee Katrina by car efficiently) makes this point clearly—even though car owners may still, falsely, see swift evacuation by car as a symbol of their own individual initiative. Jack Aiello and coauthor Lyra Stein as well as Karen M. O'Neill further show that the facile division between private initiative and the public sector does not stand up to scrutiny. As we see in the pages of this volume, economic prosperity and self-sufficiency (whether in housing or transportation) have been maintained through extraordinary federal and state government involvement. But the essays go further, arguing that these government-enabled structures (such as public transportation or the existence of highways and evacuation plans) conceal their origins—while creating the myths about individualism and initiative on one hand and dependence and vulnerability on the other.

True comprehension about the meaning and imprint of a disaster like Katrina involves thinking through causes and consequences in a sustained and committed way. The insufficient and short-lived nature of the media's and the government's engagement with Katrina brought the authors of this volume together to reflect and to continue reflecting on the storm, its prehistory, its aftermath and its lasting legacy. In recent years, as Keith Wailoo and Jeffrey Dowd show, the lessons of Katrina have largely been lost in media coverage of other disasters. Often, our fast-moving world simply fails to remember.[2] Sustained attention, however, is necessary for the collective action required to address social problems.

Although the media can be critical of government and delve into some of the hidden stories of Katrina, it mostly fails to weave these accounts into a broader narrative where we can see the political and social origins of the disaster clearly. Media coverage, when it is critical of government, can leave viewers feeling cynical and ultimately powerless concerning the possibilities of change. Equally problematic, media coverage and social commentary on Katrina frequently individualizes racism, for example, with images of black citizens denied entry to Gretna or with Kanye West's claim that "Bush doesn't care about black people." But, the essays in this volume highlight that the quest for racial justice cannot be reduced to a search for hidden bigots or uncaring politicians. It must involve an examination of the systemic problems of vulnerability and racism. Here is where sustained, multidisciplinary analysis can play an important role— by calling attention to how concrete policies in health care, transportation, and the environment lay the groundwork for disaster, and by rejecting misguided myths of poverty, race, and individualism that stand in the way of social progress.

This book is organized into four thematic parts titled "The Tangled Logic of Vulnerability," "Cultural and Psychic Legacies," " 'Starting Over' in Post-Katrina America," and "Tragedy, Recovery, and Myth." Although each section may be read as a distinct piece, together they form complementary parts of the larger story of race and vulnerability.

The first part deals with the complex and historically defined character of vulnerability. In the opening essay of part I, sociologist Karen M. O'Neill shows how past decisions contributed to the failure of the levees and to the environmental vulnerability of New Orleans in general and of the poor sections of the city in particular. Historian Mia Bay then examines black immobility during the storm through the lens of a history of race and access to transportation. Historian Keith Wailoo explores what lessons can be learned by looking closely at the physical inability of those dependent on dialysis machines to leave New Orleans. Finally, political scientist Roland Anglin suggests that the system of American federalism is itself to blame for the problems associated with Katrina.

Katrina did not have simply material or economic consequences; it also made a psychic imprint on the nation as a whole. Part 2 notes Katrina's cultural and psychic impact—particularly for black Americans who have historically endured multiple cycles of trauma and displacement. Historian Ann Fabian writes, "The dead were too visible, slipped free from all the cultural nets that help the living deal with the dead." These dead bodies floating in polluted water alongside residents stranded on overpasses and roofs cast a moral shadow over the city and the nation, Fabian argues. And such sights prompted more than one newscaster and commentator to exclaim, "This is not America." Richard Mizelle Jr. asks how New Orleans's unique cultural resources, like the jazz funeral, can be called on to rejuvenate the city. Psychologist Nancy Boyd-Franklin examines psychological stress and how the idea of "vicarious racism" may help explain a kind of "collective trauma" that many black Americans experienced in the wake of Katrina. Literary scholar Evie Shockley returns to the central images of New Orleans in another way—looking not at bodies but at depictions of "wind-wrecked, water-ravaged, molding, abandoned houses" whose omnipresence in media coverage tell a story about race, homes, and American domestic ideology.

When politicians and newscasters refer to Katrina, they often refer to "lessons learned" or ask, "Have we learned the lessons of Katrina?" In part 3, our authors explore the different aspects of recovery in post-Katrina America. Historian Keith Wailoo and sociologist Jeffrey Dowd examine the coverage of floods, fires, and a bridge collapse since Katrina in order to track how the media has constructed Katrina's meaning, what lessons have been learned and articulated in the mass media about other disasters, and what the limitations of those lessons have been. Psychologists Jack Aiello and Lyra Stein find that Hurricane Katrina "exposed a fundamental difference between private sector and public sector preparedness," and they look deeply into this divergence. William Rodgers III examines how disasters disrupt capital operations and labor markets and asks who benefits and why. Finally, sociologist Niki Dickerson ponders if life is better for those who relocated out of the poverty-stricken areas of a poor city in the state with the highest poverty rate in the country.

The book's concluding section, "Tragedy, Recovery, and Myth," takes a critical view of the mythic ideal of mobility and self-reliance, because this powerful notion of American self-sufficiency shapes the lessons we learn about the hurricane and its aftermath. Legal scholar David Troutt considers what Katrina exposed about our overdeveloped sense of self-reliance. The volume ends with an essay by the editors, which probes the lessons we must learn, as a society, not simply to recover but also to avoid another such disaster.

Understanding Katrina's imprint requires diverse perspectives and multidisciplinary analysis; it requires bringing the disturbing images not only of people but also of the nation itself into greater focus; and it requires patience and a sustained commitment to unraveling a complex story that long predates the storm itself. Collectively, the essays that follow view Katrina as a hallmark event that demonstrates how poverty and inequality arise not from the actions of unsuccessful or weak individuals but rather from an entire culture and system.

The very process of sustaining analysis and engagement with Katrina is a political gesture, and keeping public attention on the storm's impact is thus in itself fraught with difficulty. Sustained attention requires leaders' as well as policymakers' ongoing promotion of the cause, an enduring media hook that keeps a story alive, or an active and visible social movement. Sustained attention could also be maintained if it were understood that the roots of disasters grow out of interests that remain in conflict. While this last statement may seem counterintuitive, a recognition of conflicts of interests would bring into focus the tough choices between competing groups, which must be acknowledged and negotiated if we, as democratic citizens, are to choose the path ahead.

In the immediate aftermath of the storm, with two major wars under way at the time of the Katrina flooding and no desire to link an ambitious recovery program to Republican Party ideals, the party in power had little to gain from keeping Katrina alive as a call for unified national action. Instead, Republicans used the crisis to push another agenda: a critique of the failures of public housing, calls for the privatization of the public school system, concerted attempts to suspend Davis-Bacon prevailing wage laws in the name of urgently rebuilding the city, and an effort to allow well-connected private contractors like Halliburton to profit in the rebuilding process. In this context, the media have struggled to find a hook, short of anniversary coverage, to keep the story going.

What is more, no unified social movement has emerged in response to the storm. In a different context and time, the events in August and September 2005 could have produced other outcomes—not unlike the great Mississippi River flood of 1927, which, along with an agricultural depression, created the context for the rise of populist leaders like Huey Long and new federal spending and new relations between the federal government and the South. It is arguable that Katrina (seen by many as a mark of incompetence stamped on the Bush administration) contributed, along with the economic crisis, to the rise of Barack Obama. Yet, leaders aside, Katrina might have produced a more ambitious national rebuilding program, a new war on poverty, or a new civil rights movement, as some predicted.[3] However, even amid a great deal of empathy among citizens—visible through the outpouring of donations to Katrina victims—there has been no coherent and visible movement stemming from Katrina, no strong advocacy for structural economic and political changes to address America's enduring questions of class, race, and vulnerability. As we will see in many of the essays, there are powerful forces keeping the poor invisible and masking the social construction of both privilege and poverty. The term *Katrina's imprint* is meant to draw attention to, and remedy, this troubling invisibility of poverty and vulnerability in the contemporary United States.

NOTES

1. Michael Harrington, *The Other America: Poverty in the United States* (Baltimore: Penguin, 1962), 11.

2. Andreas Huyssen, *Present Pasts: Urban Palimpsests and the Politics of Memory* (Stanford, Calif.: Stanford University Press, 2003).

3. David Brooks, "The Storm after the Storm," *New York Times*, September 1, 2005, 23.

PART ONE

The Tangled Logic
of Vulnerability

1

Who Sank New Orleans?

How Engineering the River Created Environmental Injustice

KAREN M. O'NEILL

New Orleans is a special case in the story of vulnerability and environmental justice. The city lies on the hurricane coast, next to two lakes, and near the end of the immense Mississippi River. The lower third of Louisiana is made of river silt deposited over the ages. Federal river and hurricane levees have prevented river silt from depositing, causing nearly all of New Orleans's land to compact and sink below the normal water levels of the nearby Mississippi River and Lake Pontchartrain. The city must run pumping stations to remove water from its storm sewer system into city-built drainage canals even after the slightest rainstorm. Protective coastal wetlands had also been historically replenished by silt deposit. They are now deprived of silt, are crossed by canals and oil and gas pipelines, and are rapidly being washed away. Katrina's storm surge broke federal hurricane levees and the federal- and city-built floodwalls and levees along drainage canals leading to the lake, easily flooding the city. Although the massive federal levees along the Mississippi River stayed intact during Katrina, these river levees did the most to make the city subside in the first place. This chapter focuses on the origins of the federal flood control program, which built all the federal projects and which, I argue, was responsible for the policies that left the city vulnerable.[1]

Hurricane Katrina showed graphically how policy by increment—in this case, policies related to public works, flood control, and housing—harms the weakest. Public works are physical and cultural systems for ordering social life. Public works also tether us to places. Many people therefore viewed the extreme disorder after Hurricane Katrina as the failure of systems that, they assumed, were designed to ensure safety and security. But U.S. flood control was never designed with safety foremost in mind; rather, it began in the late nineteenth century as a program to promote economic development and to unify the nation. For decades, whatever public safety protections existed were limited to partial levee lines in a few cities west of the Appalachian range. Over time, the number of people living near flood-prone rivers increased dramatically, with poor African Americans and other marginalized groups often clustering in hazardous areas. Demands to improve the safety of these more recently settled lands grew, but those demands taxed a program that was created primarily to extend farming onto floodplains. Fundamentally then, the system has no mandate to assess the cumulated conditions that make some people keenly vulnerable.

The Katrina disaster reveals clearly how tensions between the historic goals of public safety and economic development have been left unresolved in the federal flood control program, primarily because within the federal system of government, legislators have little interest and limited leverage to create comprehensive, long-term plans for any area of policy. Moreover, national and state legislatures do not directly supervise the bureaucracies that administer government policies. So rather than reforming an agency's overall program when new needs emerge, legislators usually just add the new tasks to the agency's docket. As a result of these general features of the federal system, while public expectations about safety have increased, they have not been matched by coordinated policies to reduce our exposure to hazards, to protect socially essential areas that remain vulnerable, and to provide emergency services when protections fail.[2] In lieu of coordinated policies that reduce exposure and risk, a variety of government programs to build flood control works (like those described above for New Orleans) and to respond to flood emergencies have accumulated at the national, state, and local levels.

Policies like these—which grow by increment—often yield dangers that go unnoticed, and particularly harms to the weak. Indeed, a world of previously unnoticed risks became tragically evident in the wake of Katrina. Calling attention to unnoticed harms is the purpose of the environmental justice movement.[3] Researchers of environmental injustice in the United States typically take two approaches: making statistical comparisons to see whether some groups experience more injuries than others do, or studying individual cases of environmental harm to trace how patterns of injustice develop. Statistical studies have not found consistent results, but they tend to show that some social groups are disproportionately exposed to environmental hazards. Case studies find that harms almost always result from the interaction of long-term structural and institutional causes rather than from targeted acts of overt racism or class bias.[4]

Katrina therefore reveals a fundamental tension. Providing for public safety in these settings requires legal or informal limitations on land use, constant vigilance, and readiness to respond to emergencies throughout settled areas. Providing for economic development does not. Unable to resolve this tension, the federal flood control program has in some ways made us less safe. The program focuses on engineering our rivers to control storm flows rather than on avoiding settlement on low-lying lands. The program's success so far is that while more people now live in floodplains, few die from river and rainstorm flooding. Yet another break in a major levee on a highly engineered river could suddenly push fast-flowing water into one of our cities with explosive force far greater than Katrina brought to New Orleans.

Taking up a theme that Roland Anglin discusses in detail at the end of this section of the book, this chapter presents a historically grounded case study, an analysis of how, over many decades, *incrementalism* in policies made the Gulf Coast, and especially New Orleans, vulnerable to Katrina and made poor African Americans in the city especially vulnerable. Each of the relevant policies affecting settlement and safety, ranging from emergency rescue to public housing, grew by increment. The accumulated effect was to concentrate poor African Americans in locations at risk for flooding and, as William Rodgers's essay explains further, to render them unable to adequately respond to the hurricane and to rebuild their lives. The intersection of race and physical vulnerability produced by river and coastal engineering and settlement policies has received little attention in post-Katrina commentary. To illuminate how the Katrina debacle was politically and physically possible, I describe the social origins of the federal flood control program, administered by the U.S. Army Corps of Engineers.

Race, Federal Relations, and Development
of the Lower Mississippi River

When the United States made the Louisiana Purchase in 1803, it opened a new round of debates about the proper nature of the union and its states, centering on how the new territories would be developed and integrated. Under United States rule, New Orleans came to depend on upstream agricultural and industrial economies staffed by family farmers, merchants, and industrial workers in the North, and slaves, sharecroppers, tenants, and merchants in the South. Resource politics and the racial formation of the northern and southern states shaped these regional economies and set up some of the conflicts leading to the Civil War. Agricultural growth along the lower Mississippi in particular depended on river flood control, which allowed planters to drain and farm rich bottomlands.[5] Two centuries of politics about race and resources helped create that agricultural base, influenced settlement patterns in the Mississippi Valley, dominated relations between valley states and the federal government, and laid the ground for the Hurricane Katrina catastrophe.[6]

From the 1820s onward, development advocates from the lower Mississippi Valley worked to make the local and regional troubles of river navigation and flooding into national concerns.[7] For European settler elites in the West, one unifying and broad cause was to gain federal development aid that would allow their new regions to compete with the long-settled Northeast in the emerging national market.[8] The U.S. Supreme Court had defined a broad scope for the federal government's domestic powers in an 1824 ruling that state governments, private toll-takers, and steamboat monopolies could not restrict free access to interstate rivers. Following on this major interpretation of the Constitution's interstate commerce clause, Congress passed a bill requiring the U.S. Army Corps of Engineers to ensure that the rivers were physically accessible for navigation.[9] From the start of this national navigation improvement program, western members of Congress complained that most aid went to the Northeast.[10]

Regional competition for river, railroad, and other forms of development aid persisted. By the 1850s, the Whig Party, with its emphasis on nationally integrated systems of infrastructure rather than piecemeal approaches, had shriveled in the heat of debates about slavery and southern power. Leaders and voters from northern states aligned increasingly with the Republican Party, while those from southern states aligned increasingly with the Democrats. In the late 1850s, northern Republicans asserted their dominance in the national government by passing batches of bills for river improvement and other economic measures that benefited the North, even as southern states threatened to secede from the Union.[11]

The Civil War itself harmed the Mississippi River's navigation channel and the small levee systems that landowners and their state-chartered levee districts had managed to build. Most of the damage occurred because the corps suspended channel clearing and because local work on levees was neglected by planters who took their agricultural slaves to war.[12] After the war, river advocates and politicians from the lower Mississippi Valley argued that it was now the federal government's responsibility to restore the navigation channel and to begin providing flood control aid to reunify the nation. The governor of Louisiana, J. Madison Wells, even argued that "the destruction of slavery" and other war losses had made landowners unable to maintain their own levees that protected crops—crops that were vital to the nation's economy and, Wells argued, vital to those slaves whom northern armies had freed. Yet most African Americans freed from slavery lived in undesirable locations. Along the Mississippi River, these included disease-ridden areas of port cities and flood-prone rural bottomlands that became available for farming once flood control levees had been built.[13]

Advocates from the Mississippi Valley allied with development advocates from the far West seeking irrigation and flood control aid. Flood control activists from the Sacramento Valley in northern California complained that gold mining in the Sierras had financed the Union's armies in the Civil War but had left farm fields in the valley below damaged from heavy deposits of mining debris. River advocates from the Mississippi and Sacramento valleys began to make similar arguments—that war (and the gold-mining to finance it) prevented their regions from integrating into the nation and the national market. The federal government therefore had an obligation to compensate them by reengineering their rivers.[14]

As regions west of the Appalachian range gained population, western river advocates won federal aid step by step, including navigation projects, engineering studies of flood problems, and eventually aid for levee building. In the late nineteenth century, northern Republicans still won elections by reminding voters that southerners had provoked the war, making it unthinkable to openly advocate aid to benefit former slave owners. It was also politically questionable to promote federal aid that would increase the value of private land. Yet by the 1870s, northern politicians allowed for accommodations of the southern elites. Congress quietly approved levee repair along the lower Mississippi by defining it as part of the corps's "navigation" improvement program.[15] The backdoor beginnings of the flood control program made it easier than it might otherwise have been for white planters to use levees to affirm their local power by extending farming onto the wettest lands along the river, such as the Mississippi-Yazoo Delta. Tenancy and sharecropping came to dominate these areas, transferring most of the economic risk of farming, including flood risk, onto these mainly African American laborers.[16]

At the turn of the century, Mississippi and California flood control advocates created a joint national lobby and public awareness campaign. They pressed members of Congress from these two valleys to focus intently on vote trading to advance their cause. The main flood control lobby organization from the lower Mississippi led the drive, convincing members of Congress to trade votes and other favors to pass the first official flood control act in 1917, for the Mississippi and Sacramento rivers. Support from the Illinois delegation, upstream on the Mississippi River, apparently led the way to the 1928 Flood Control Act, passed in response to the still-unsurpassed floods throughout the Mississippi Valley in 1927. The 1928 act promised to wholly remake the Sacramento and Mississippi rivers, and it became the model for the nationwide program of flood control passed in 1936.[17]

The flood control program and the more recent coastal protection program have been built over decades, project by project, by bills passed every few years. Critics have complained that Congress's control over the lists of projects in those bills inclines members to spread program money to many legislative districts rather than setting priorities to protect the country's most vulnerable sites. Some critics see the Corps of Engineers as complicit with this approach, but others view the corps as limited in its ability to guide project approval or to prompt review of the overall performance of protections on any given river.[18]

Federalism also means that Congress and the Corps of Engineers do not fully control the way federal projects are built. The corps parcels out levee building to local contractors whose mistakes may delay construction or lead to levee failure. State governments and local levee districts coordinate with the corps and its contractors, pay a share of project costs, and maintain the federal levees. Local disputes over land rights or problems in raising local or state funds may slow or block federal projects.

Independent projects by local governments and private landowners further complicate river development and disaster response. Local governments and levee districts supplement federal projects by constructing local protections that are seldom built to federal standards. For New Orleans, such local projects include the city's pump systems, nearly all of which failed during Katrina. In addition, private owners drain their farmlands into ditches that feed into rivers, and municipalities add their storm water, further stressing federal levees on major waterways downstream.

The federal government asserts little direct control over land use in areas that remain vulnerable to flooding—for example, setting no limits on building in floodplains after completion of nearby federal levees. Local planning and zoning boards then make thousands of decisions each year to develop lots, gradually reshaping the floodplains and affecting exposure to flood hazards in unpredictable ways. Homebuyers and renters choose housing and business space with little information about flooding hazards. The federal government and many municipalities have promoted floodplain management since the midtwentieth century to coordinate decisions about land use and flood protection, but its effectiveness is limited because it was adopted only after engineering had already remade nearly all of our major rivers.[19]

Why Were African Americans in New Orleans So Vulnerable?

Vulnerability in New Orleans is not a simple matter. Media accounts just after the hurricane occasionally captured certain features and causes of the city's vulnerability (its below-sea-level proximity and its precarious place on the Gulf shore), but most reporters had trouble representing the complex interaction of human engineering, environmental constraints, racial and class segregation, and federal powers that the essays in this volume examine. Add the lack of social and economic resources available to impoverished African Americans in New Orleans, and we see why so many of them ended up in their attics or on their roofs waiting for help after the hurricane.

Although New Orleanians have constantly renegotiated the borders between black, white, Creole, Cajun, and many other identities, even in this historically tolerant city, African Americans (defined broadly here) have at times been disadvantaged through segregation. From the early nineteenth century, segregation laws and housing markets limited free African Americans and slaves in New Orleans to specific locations and restricted their movements, although less so than in other southern cities. The city's coordinated drainage and sewerage program began in the 1890s, eventually benefiting existing African American as well as white neighborhoods. By the 1930s, however, Jim Crow policies meant that swampy city lands opened to development by the drainage program would be segregated, with new African American areas typically being low and susceptible to flooding.[20]

A range of nationwide practices also structured a segregated housing market. From the early twentieth century, private market appraisals gave the least risky ratings to mortgages in all white, middle-class neighborhoods with single-family houses. It is unclear whether federal home loan programs contributed substantially to these private market practices, but those federal loans and loan guarantees that did aid African Americans apparently had little effect on overall patterns of segregation.[21] Federal highway spending from the 1950s onward further encouraged the spread of residential development in the suburbs. White flight in response to the civil rights and Black Power movements and school desegregation dramatically remade many mixed New Orleans neighborhoods into majority African American areas, including the Ninth Ward.[22] The civil rights era yielded some protections for African Americans, including increased financing for various government housing programs, but the long-term toleration and even encouragement of segregation in federal loan policies and public housing policies had lasting effects on settlement patterns.[23] These federal policies were associated with the overall economic decline of most large cities. Government redevelopment programs for cities yielded few benefits to African American residents and indeed often displaced them from neighborhoods declared blighted.

Despite the many problems, low-income African American residents continued to express exceptionally strong attachments to New Orleans. An impressive number of low-income African Americans in the city managed to own houses, often self-built, and many managed to pass them down to their descendants.[24] As well, many residents who moved into segregated public housing rental apartments built in the 1950s (nearly always on flood-prone lands) saw them as better than the units available to them on the market, and they built extensive social ties there.[25] Sadly, the obligations of mortgage payments, even on houses destroyed by the hurricane, now limit the options and choices of low-income homeowners.[26] Outsiders who wonder why residents "chose" housing susceptible to flooding disregard the legacy of laws and hostility that excluded most African Americans from the surrounding suburbs. They also overlook the economic and social value of these residences, such as the social networks these areas provide for some of the poorest New Orleanians.

Effects of the Storm

Fortress defense—the principle on which the levee system was based—requires that all walls remain unbreached. On August 29, 2005, the storm's surge from the east broke levees along two corps shipping canals near Lake Borgne—the Mississippi River Gulf Outlet and the Intercoastal Waterway—and wind and water from Lake Pontchartrain broke floodwalls along the Industrial Canal, London Avenue Canal, and Seventeenth Avenue Canal. Drainage pumps that lost power or cooling water, or that were untended, were unable to pump out rain that fell directly on Jefferson Parish and elsewhere. Pre-storm predictions used for system designs were wrong in many ways. Failures occurred at the points that were weakest because of design or construction faults or differences in the underlying soil structures.[27]

Coordination of an effective emergency response to such a storm would have been difficult for any city. As Roland Anglin discusses in his essay, it was immeasurably more difficult for New Orleans given its economically weak base, the lack of an internal stable coalition of government, business, and civil society groups, and tenuous relationships with state and federal partners.[28] The Federal Emergency Management Agency and state and local agencies did not manage to implement the plans they had on the shelf. The city's evacuation plan, such as it was, depended on residents driving themselves away from town, which, Mia Bay explains in the next chapter, was not possible for the many poor residents who had no cars.[29]

Objective measures of social vulnerability to disasters show why the storm's effects were worst in New Orleans. Outside New Orleans, whites actually suffered a greater share of the damages than African Americans did. Inside New Orleans, floodwaters did not select by race or class, but members of disadvantaged groups had higher odds of living in damaged areas.[30] There, renters, African Americans, the poor, women, and the elderly suffered disproportionately and had fewer social and economic resources than others for coping.[31] A post-storm survey of New Orleans residents found that low-income African Americans were most likely to have stayed during the hurricane and were least able to evacuate on their own once it hit.[32] The misfortune of poor African Americans in particular is that the exchange relationships that had supported their daily living before Katrina could not provide what they needed most during and after the storm—cars to escape the flood, savings to restart or rebuild, and access to social networks that could provide them high-paying jobs.

Isolation, Invisibility, and the Accumulation of Unnoticed Harms

In New Orleans, Hurricane Katrina broke the social order that the levees had long represented. For years, scientists had warned about the system's many vulnerabilities, activists had warned that the area was in grave environmental decline, and social scientists had warned that many residents would not be able or willing to evacuate.[33] Ordinary people watching the storm scenes on television knew something else, that an implied promise had been broken. The sum of government actions across policy areas and at all levels of the federal system had allowed and even encouraged people to build near the coast and on floodplains and had contributed to land subsidence and the decline of environmental functions. Populations located near most coastal areas in the United States had increased dramatically in the twentieth century. Hadn't government actions encouraging these developments implied that this pattern of growth was safe?

Placing safety above economic development as the goal for the Corps of Engineers's river flood control and coastal protection programs would require reconsidering basic assumptions for the entire engineered system. One far-reaching question about the river program would be whether we should build long miles of levee lines to protect upriver farmland and warehouses, a policy that increases the water flowing past populated downriver areas. Questions for the coastal program would be whether we should pay to replenish recreational beaches and allow building on lands repeatedly devastated by storms. Over the years, big cities have made the most powerful demands for public safety protections. Emergency responders, scientists, and floodplain managers, who have even less political pull than cities do, have attempted to coordinate existing hazard and disaster policies. They receive only occasional aid for this behind-the-scenes work. As a result, the response to Hurricane Katrina was led by a fragmented set of organizations working around the margins of overstretched engineering programs that try to promote both economic development and public safety.

In the social catastrophe of Katrina, we can see the limitations that are designed into our federal system and that incline politicians toward incremental decision making. Hazard policies and disaster response preparations are divided among agencies that are at best loosely coupled. Several values are expressed most strongly in this system. One value is to promote economic development. Another is to protect private property rights, including an implied right to develop the land as the owner sees fit. A third is to preserve local prerogative to approve the development of private land and the use of police powers in emergencies, as bulwarks against the concentration of power at the central government. A strongly centralized government would not necessarily be able to enact more effective policies. These observations simply highlight the weaknesses that our particular system has produced.

On August 29, 2005, we witnessed the consequences of a nation that had no coherent policy for protecting the most socially isolated and disadvantaged people in our society. The rhetoric of nineteenth-century river advocates was self-serving, but they were correct to state that public works define the nation. The debate and government action in the years following the storm has not been encouraging. Rebuilding the levees alone will not do. Creating more environmentally sound infrastructure at this late date may be not enough to revitalize the region and its people. Even if it would be enough, there seems to be little political will to take the most obvious steps in that direction. And in the meantime, the poor, mostly African American citizens and now displaced residents of New Orleans—the most obvious victims of incrementalism—continue to live with harms that others do not notice.

ACKNOWLEDGMENT

A version of this chapter, in substantially different form, appeared in the journal *Southern Cultures*, which has kindly allowed me to include that material here.

NOTES

1. See John M. Barry, *Rising Tide: The Great Mississippi Flood of 1927 and How It Changed America* (New York: Simon and Schuster, 1997); Craig E. Colten, "Basin Street Blues: Drainage and Environmental Equity in New Orleans, 1890–1930," *Journal of Historical Geography* 28, no. 2 (2002): 237–257; Major D. O. Elliott, *The Improvement of the Lower Mississippi River for Flood Control and Navigation* (Vicksburg, Miss.: U.S. Waterways Experiment Station, Corps of Engineers, U.S. Army, 1932); Andrew A. Humphreys and Henry L. Abbot, "Report upon the Physics and Hydraulics of the Mississippi River" (Washington, D.C.: United States War Department, 1861); John McPhee, "Atchafalaya," in *The Control of Nature* (New York: Farrar Straus Giroux, 1986).

2. Martin Reuss, "The Development of American Water Resources: Planners, Politicians, and Constitutional Interpretation," in *Managing Water Resources Past and Present*, ed. Julie Trottier and Paul Slack (Oxford: Oxford University Press, 2004).

3. Robert Bullard, *Dumping in Dixie: Race, Class, and Environmental Quality* (Boulder, Colo.: Westview Press, 1990).

4. For example, Eric J. Krieg, "Race and Environmental Justice in Buffalo, NY: A Zip Code and Historical Analysis of Ecological Hazards," *Society and Natural Resources* 18 (2005): 199–213; Robin Saha and Paul Mohai, "Historical Context and Hazardous Waste Facility Siting: Understanding Temporal Patterns in Michigan," *Social Problems* 52, no. 4 (2005): 618–648; Christine A. Bevc, Brent K. Marshall, and J. Steven Picou, "Environmental Justice and Toxic Exposure: Toward a Spatial Model of Physical Health and Psychological Well-Being," *Social Science Research* 36, no. 1 (2007): 48–67.

5. Bottomlands are low-lying lands near rivers—areas that are typically prone to flooding.

6. This account of the origins of the federal flood control program is based on my book *Rivers by Design: State Power and the Origins of U.S. Flood Control* (Durham, N.C.: Duke University Press, 2006).

7. See, for example, St. Louis Chamber of Commerce, *Proceedings of the St. Louis Chamber of Commerce, in Relation to the Improvement of the Navigation of the Mississippi River and Its Principal Tributaries and the St. Louis Harbor: With a Statement Submitted by A. B. Chambers to the Chamber* (St. Louis: St. Louis Chamber of Commerce, 1842); Barry, *Rising Tide*, 34.

8. Sean Wilentz, "Society, Politics, and the Market Revolution, 1815–1848," in *The New American History*, ed. Eric Foner (Philadelphia: Temple University Press, 1990).

9. Todd Shallat, *Structures in the Stream: Water, Science, and the Rise of the U.S. Army Corps of Engineers* (Austin: University of Texas Press, 1994).

10. River conventions were the key venue. The largest was in 1847: *Harbor and River Convention [of 1847] Chicago, Memorial to the Congress of the United States of the Executive Committee of the*

Convention Held at Chicago, July 5, 1847: With an Abstract of the Convention, on the Improvement of Rivers and Harbors. Presented to Congress, June 1848 (Albany, N.Y.: Harbor and River Convention, Chicago, 1848).

11. Richard Franklin Bensel, *Sectionalism and American Political Development, 1880–1980* (Madison: University of Wisconsin Press, 1984); Morton Keller, *Affairs of State: Public Life in Late Nineteenth Century America* (Cambridge, Mass.: Belknap Press of Harvard University Press, 1977); C. Vann Woodward, *Reunion and Reaction: The Compromise of 1877 and the End of Reconstruction* (Boston: Little Brown, 1966); Paul W. Gates, *Agriculture and the Civil War* (New York: Alfred A. Knopf, 1965); Richard Franklin Bensel, *Yankee Leviathan: The Origins of Central State Authority in America, 1859–1877* (Cambridge: Cambridge University Press, 1990).

12. Elliott, *The Improvement of the Lower Mississippi River for Flood Control and Navigation*; Robert W. Harrison, *Levee Districts and Levee Building in Mississippi: A Study of State and Local Efforts to Control Mississippi River Floods* (Washington, D.C.: Bureau of Agricultural Economics, USDA, Delta Council, The Board of Mississippi Levee Commissioners, Board of Levee Commissioners for the Yazoo-Mississippi Delta and Mississippi Agricultural Experiment Station, Cooperating with the Bureau of Agricultural Economics, U.S. Department of Agriculture, 1951).

13. J. Maddison [*sic*] Wells, *The National Importance of Rebuilding and Repairing the Levees, on the Banks of the Mississippi . . .* (N.p., n.d., c. 1860s).

14. George Ruble Woolfolk, *The Cotton Regency: The Northern Merchants and Reconstruction, 1865–1880* (New York: Bookman Associates, 1958); Wells, *The National Importance of Rebuilding and Repairing the Levees*; Harrison, *Levee Districts and Levee Building in Mississippi*; Union Merchants' Exchange of St. Louis, *Report of the Committee on Improvement of the Mississippi River and Tributaries: St. Louis, 15th December, 1865* (St. Louis: Union Merchants' Exchange of St. Louis, 1865?).

15. Charles A. Camillo and Matthew T. Pearcy, *Upon Their Shoulders: A History of the Mississippi River Commission from Its Inception through the Advent of the Modern Mississippi River and Tributaries Project* (Vicksburg, Miss.: Mississippi River Commission, 2004); H. B. Ferguson, *History of the Improvement of the Lower Mississippi River for Flood Control and Navigation, 1932–1939* (Vicksburg, Miss.: Mississippi River Commission, 1940); U.S. Congress, *Congressional Record*, 64th Cong., 1st sess. (May 10, 1916).

16. Harrison, *Levee Districts and Levee Building in Mississippi*; Barry, *Rising Tide*, Charles S. Aiken, "The Decline of Sharecropping in the Lower Mississippi River Valley," *Geoscience and Man* 19 (1978): 161–165.

17. Matthew T. Pearcy, "After the Flood: A History of the 1928 Flood Control Act," *Journal of the Illinois State Historical Society* 95, no. 2 (2002): 172–201; Arthur DeWitt Frank, *The Development of the Federal Program of Flood Control on the Mississippi River* (1930; repr., New York: AMS Press, 1968).

18. Shallat, *Structures in the Stream*.

19. Raymond J. Burby, "Hurricane Katrina and the Paradoxes of Government Disaster Policy: Bringing About Wise Governmental Decisions for Hazardous Areas," *Annals of the American Academy of Political and Social Science* 604 (2006): 171–191; Jamie W. Moore and Dorothy P. Moore, *The Army Corps of Engineers and the Evolution of Federal Flood Plain Management Policy* (Boulder, Colo.: Institute of Behavioral Science, University of Colorado, 1989).

20. Roger A. Fischer, "Racial Segregation in Ante Bellum New Orleans," *American Historical Review* 74, no. 3 (1969): 926–937; Craig E. Colten, "Vulnerability and Place: Flat Land and Uneven Risk in New Orleans," *American Anthropologist* 108, no. 4 (2006): 731–734; Colten, "Basin Street Blues"; C. Vann Woodward, *The Strange Career of Jim Crow* (New York: Oxford University Press, 2002).

21. Kenneth T. Jackson, "Race, Ethnicity, and Real Estate Appraisal: The Home Owners Loan Corporation and the Federal Housing Administration," *Journal of Urban History* 6, no. 4 (1980): 419–452; Amy E. Hillier, "Redlining and the Home Owners Loan Corporation," *Journal of Urban History* 29, no. 4 (2003): 394–420.

22. Rachel Breunlin and Helen A. Regis, "Putting the Ninth Ward on the Map: Race, Place, and Transformation in Desire, New Orleans," *American Anthropologist* 108, no. 4 (2006): 744–764.

23. Chris Bonastia, "Hedging His Bets: Why Nixon Killed HUD's Desegregation Efforts," *Social Science History* 28, no. 1 (2004): 19–52; Arnold R. Hirsch, "'Containment' on the Home Front: Race and Federal Housing Policy from the New Deal to the Cold War," *Journal of Urban History* 26, no. 2 (2000): 158–189.

24. John R. Logan, "The Impact of Katrina: Race and Class in Storm-Damaged Neighborhoods," available at http://www.54.brown.edu/katrina/report.pdf.

25. Breunlin and Regis, "Putting the Ninth Ward on the Map."

26. James R. Elliott and Jeremy Pais, "Race, Class, and Hurricane Katrina: Social Differences in Human Responses to Disaster," *Social Science Research* 35 (2006): 295–321.

27. Dan Swenson and Bob Marshall, "Flash Flood: Hurricane Katrina's Inundation of New Orleans, August 29, 2005—Interactive Graphic," *Times-Picayune*, May 14, 2006; Interagency Performance Evaluation Task Force, *Performance Evaluation of the New Orleans and Southeast Louisiana Hurricane Protection System: Interim Final Report of the Interagency Performance Evaluation Task Force* (New Orleans: U.S. Army Corps of Engineers, 2007).

28. See also Peter Burns and Matthew O. Thomas, "The Failure of the Nonregime: How Katrina Exposed New Orleans as a Regimeless City," *Urban Affairs Review* 41, no. 4 (2006): 517–527.

29. Colten, "Vulnerability and Place"; Citizens for Responsibility and Ethics in Washington, *The Best Laid Plans: The Story of How the Government Ignored Its Own Gulf Coast Hurricane Plans* (Washington, D.C.: CREW, 2007).

30. Logan, "The Impact of Katrina."

31. Colten, "Vulnerability and Place"; Susan L. Cutter and Christopher T. Emrich, "Moral Hazard, Social Catastrophe: The Changing Face of Vulnerability along the Hurricane Coasts," *Annals of the American Academy of Political and Social Science* 604 (2006): 102–112; Logan, "The Impact of Katrina."

32. Elliott and Pais, "Race, Class, and Hurricane Katrina."

33. Shirley Laska, "What if Hurricane Ivan Had Not Missed New Orleans?" *Natural Hazards Observer* 29, no. 2 (2004): http://www.colorado.edu/hazards/o/archives/2004/novo4/novo4c.html; Ivor van Heerden and Mike Bryan, *The Storm: What Went Wrong and Why during Hurricane Katrina—the inside Story from One Louisiana Scientist* (New York: Viking, 2006).

2

Invisible Tethers

Transportation and Discrimination
in the Age of Katrina

MIA BAY

New Orleans came into being as a transportation hub. Located between the Mississippi River and Lake Pontchartrain, the city first took shape as a trading post at the point of portage between these two bodies of water. There, goods and people traveling along the inland waterways of the continent's longest river could connect with Atlantic trade routes that began in the Gulf of Mexico. The city, formed around this intersection of waterways, became one the continent's primary transfer points for both domestic and transatlantic goods. Founded by French and Scottish entrepreneurs in 1718, its initial growth was propelled by the fur trade. But by the antebellum era, the fur trade had gone the way of the beaver, and New Orleans became better known for its trade in people. Acquired by the United States in 1803, when Jefferson bought the vast territory known as Louisiana from the French, the city was already "one of the principal slave markets for North America."[1] New Orleans became still more important to the continent's slave trade after 1808, when the United States withdrew from the international slave trade. The domestic trade, which was centered in New Orleans, boomed in consequence, transforming the former trading post into the nation's second-largest port city.

Throughout the antebellum era, New Orleans's slave market was at the center of the domestic slave trade that sustained the expansion of the plantation South and inspired the slave spiritual "Many Thousands Gone." A mournful dirge, the song commemorates the vast, involuntary migration of enslaved African Americans, sold from the old slave states in the upper South to new states and territories on the lower South's expanding cotton frontier, usually via New Orleans. In short, the city was the place where many slaves who had been "sold down the river" met their new owners.

After emancipation, the waters of the Mississippi no longer carried black people deeper into slavery. Emancipation marked the beginning of the end of

New Orleans's status as a premier port city. In the wake of the Civil War, not only was it a slave market no more, but the waterways that had made New Orleans a commercial hub began to lose their significance as a national network of railways took shape. Whereas black travelers aboard antebellum steamboats had often traveled against their will, shackled together in slave coffles bound for the New Orleans auction block, with emancipation, black access to common carriers became newly circumscribed.

But the movement of peoples in and around New Orleans continued to be shaped both by race and by water. The war's end brought attempts by white employers across the South to restrict the movements of the freed people by way of vagrancy laws and other black codes that mimicked the system of bondage that once held black workers in place. But Reconstruction came early in Louisiana, which fell under Union control in 1862; as a result, freed people there never experienced the worst excesses of the postemancipation black codes. Still, African Americans in the state never achieved sustained equal access to transportation, a situation that arguably continues to this day. Consequently, New Orleans—Louisiana's transportation hub—has been a battleground for African American challenges to discrimination on common carriers from emancipation onward, and into the era of Katrina.

The Power of Locomotion: *Plessy* as a Precedent for Katrina

Entirely excluded from the New Orleans streetcar system as emancipation dawned, African Americans fought for access to the transportation network that served their city during the post–Civil War era—with mixed success. New Orleans's municipal streetcars were desegregated in 1867 and remained legally integrated until 1902.[2] But African Americans never won unrestricted access to the city's waterways or railroads. Black plantation owner Josephine DeCuir's 1870s challenge to a New Orleans steamboat company that barred her from occupying "a cabin specially set apart for white people" marked the limits of de jure transportation equity in postemancipation Louisiana. Initially upheld under Louisiana's Civil Rights Act of 1869, DeCuir's case was overturned by the United States Supreme Court in the 1878 decision *Hall v. DeCuir* on the grounds that Louisiana had no power to regulate carriers engaged in interstate commerce. With this decision, one commentator notes, "the Supreme Court began the legal journey toward *Civil Rights Cases* of 1883," which ruled that although the Fourteenth Amendment's enforcement provisions allowed the federal government to outlaw racial discriminatory measures passed by state and local governments, Congress had no power "to prohibit discrimination by private individuals."[3]

Such decisions combined to eviscerate much of the Fourteenth Amendment's promise of "equal protection" for black civil rights, setting the stage for *Plessy v. Ferguson*—the most famous of all the segregation cases. Like the *DeCuir* case, *Plessy* was a New Orleans transportation case. The ruling that enshrined the Jim Crow South's legal doctrine of separate-but-equal originated in 1890 when Homer Plessy, a New Orleans shoemaker of Creole ancestry, was jailed for sitting in the "white" car of the East Louisiana Railroad. Only one-eighth black, Plessy challenged Louisiana's 1890 separate car law on behalf of the New Orleans Citizen's Council, an African American civil rights organization whose members asked Plessy to lead their test case on account of his mixed ancestry. Their hope was that Plessy's predominately white ancestry and Caucasian appearance might complicate and undermine the legislative logic behind the separate car laws adopted by Louisiana and other states in the wake of Reconstruction.

Purely race-based, these laws required all blacks to travel in railroad compartments reserved for the colored. Separate but in no way equal, the colored cars were rail compartments that in the years prior to the emergence of segregation on the railroads had traditionally been reserved for second-class passengers who wished to smoke. Crowded and noisy, and lacking amenities such as upholstered seats and water closets, these cars rode directly behind the engine, exposing the passengers who traveled in them to the soot and noise it generated. Moreover, they also continued to accommodate smokers of all races, even as they became the only place where black people were allowed to travel.

However, neither the Supreme Court of Louisiana nor the Supreme Court of the United States took notice of conditions in the colored cars or Homer Plessy's mixed racial ancestry when they upheld the lower court's ruling against him. John Howard Ferguson, the Louisiana state court judge, had held that the state was free to regulate railways that operated only in Louisiana. Returning to the same issue, the United States Supreme Court affirmed his ruling, insisting that segregated transportation posed no challenge to the African American civil rights protected by the Fourteenth Amendment. The Court held that "the object of the [Fourteenth A]mendment was undoubtedly to enforce the absolute equality of the two races before the law, but in the nature of things it could not have been intended to abolish distinctions based upon color, or to enforce social, as distinguished from political equality, or a commingling of the two races upon terms unsatisfactory to either."[4]

A landmark decision most known today for its applications beyond transportation, *Plessy v. Ferguson* provided the legal basis for separate schools, restaurants, theaters, hospitals, cemeteries, and public facilities of all kinds from 1896 through 1954, when the legal doctrine of separate but equal was overturned by the Supreme Court's *Brown v. Board of Education* decision. However, in wake of recent events in New Orleans, the issues involved in *Plessy*'s support of segregated transportation retain their relevance and are worth revisiting. For, despite the broad applications that would shape its subsequent history, *Plessy* ultimately turned on the issue of public access to transportation, which Justice John Marshall Harlan, the sole dissenter on the *Plessy* verdict, discussed with great eloquence. Railroads, he noted, were public "highways." Although privately owned, they served the public and exercised public functions, as demonstrated by state legislatures' use of the public-spirited right of eminent domain to seize land for the construction of railroad tracks. "The right to eminent domain nowhere justifies taking property for private use," he emphasized. Accordingly, Harlan reasoned, all citizens should have equal rights to the use of the railroads as a matter of civil rights. "Personal Liberty," he maintained, citing Black's *Constitutional Law*, "consists of the power of locomotion, or changing situation, or removing one's person to whatsoever places one's inclination may direct."[5]

Harlan's words are newly resonant in the aftermath of Hurricane Katrina, where we saw a tremendous failure in the power of personal locomotion that was largely defined by race. Katrina's illustration of persistent and pervasive racial inequities regarding transportation in the United States suggests how little this nation has really traveled since *Plessy*. Described by some as a wake-up call about racial inequality in America, Katrina left behind—in the Superdome, stranded on the rooftops of their homes, and paddling through the waters that flooded New Orleans—a group of residents who were overwhelmingly black.[6] Also among those unable to evacuate were prisoners, the elderly, and disabled people, both black and white—many of whom did not survive. Indeed, the old and the sick number prominently among Katrina's fatalities—for obvious reasons.[7] What unifies this group is their social status as immobile people, a status overcome during emergencies only if adequate money and planning are in place. But what explains that race, rather than age and physical fragility, was the common factor that united the vast majority of those who remained in the city after Katrina struck?

Of the 270,000 Katrina survivors stuck in New Orleans, 93 percent were black. And those left behind shared characteristics that are often unevenly distributed by race. They were predominately poor and unskilled: 77 percent had a high school education or less, 68 percent had neither money in the bank nor a useable credit card, and 57 percent had total household incomes of less than $20,000 per year. Poverty is one of the major reasons why many of the evacuees did not manage to leave before the storm. They lacked the resources to either travel or support themselves once they relocated. Moreover, the evacuees also tended to share one characteristic closely related to both their racial and economic demographics: 55 percent had no car or other way to evacuate.[8] In this respect, Hurricane Katrina's victims were not unique to New Orleans. Although no longer legally prohibited from traveling freely on the nation's "public highways," like their segregation era counterparts, many contemporary African Americans both in New Orleans and elsewhere experience a similar restriction on their mobility, largely as a consequence of low levels of car ownership and a deficient public transportation system.

Access to Transportation

Across the nation, African Americans are about three times more likely to lack a car than whites. Latinos come in second when it comes to carlessness—they are two and a half times more likely to own no vehicle. The racial shape of this disparity becomes clear when one looks at the statistics: only 7 percent of white families in the United States own no vehicle, as compared with 21 percent of black households, 17 percent of Latino households, 15 percent of Native American households, and 13 percent of Asian American households—and disparities with whites are even greater in urban areas. Across the nation, people of color are also less able to rely on the cars they do own for longer trips, as might be required during emergencies like evacuation. Their cars are usually significantly older and cheaper than those owned by whites. Stereotypes about African Americans favoring Cadillacs not withstanding, cars owned by blacks and Latinos have median values in the $5,000 range, while the value of cars owned by white family households averages well over $12,000.[9] Meanwhile, the many blacks and Latinos who own no car are still worse off, as automobile owners typically have better access to employment, health care, affordable housing, and other necessities.[10] More to the point, as Katrina demonstrated, in a disaster, access to a car can be a matter of life or death.

This is especially true in urban areas such as New Orleans, where people of color constitute a larger portion of the population than they do in the country as whole. According to the 2000 U.S. Census, people of color make up 30 percent of the nation's population, but 73 percent of the population in New Orleans. In the counties affected by Hurricanes Rita, Katrina, and Wilma in 2005, blacks and Latinos made up 24 percent and 14 percent of the carless households, respectively, whereas only 7 percent of white households lacked a car.[11] These statistics acquire real urgency in the case of disasters such as the hurricanes of 2005. Unlike the citizens of nations such as Germany, Japan, Holland, and Britain, all of which have fairly comprehensive public transportation systems in place, Americans who have no access to cars are carless in a society where an automobile is often crucial to both daily life and emergency transportation.

The stranding of African Americans in New Orleans, then, can be read through the intersection of economics and racial discrimination. Although urban dwellers in metropolitan areas with effective public transportation, like New York City, sometimes choose not to own automobiles as a matter of convenience, not owning a car is inconvenient in many other American cities. The infrastructure of the highway informs the perpetuation of America as a nation obsessed with cars and car ownership. As a result, in the Big Easy, as in most of the nation's urban areas, "public transit is considered a mode of last resort or a novelty for tourists and special events. Most middle-class residents seldom use public transit and so have little reason to support it. As a result, service quality is minimal, and poorly integrated into the overall transport system."[12]

African Americans, however, depend on public transportation despite its many limitations. For low-income African Americans in New Orleans and elsewhere, the economic challenges posed by car ownership and American car culture are only compounded by the expensive and exclusionary forms of discrimination that attend virtually every economic transaction required to buy and maintain an automobile. African Americans routinely pay more for cars of similar value than whites. Though no research group has yet produced a national study of this, a 1996 class action suit against an Atlanta-area car dealership revealed that the dealership routinely made between two and seven times as much profit on cars sold to African Americans as compared with vehicles sold to whites.[13] Moreover, broader evidence from a study performed by economists Ian Ayres and Peter Siegelman suggests that such practices are not unusual. Audits of the car prices offered to more than three hundred pairs of trained testers dispatched to negotiate with Chicago-area car dealerships produced final price offers in which black males were asked to pay $1,100 more than white males for identical vehicles, while the prices offered to black and white women exceeded those offered to white men by $410 and $92, respectively.[14]

Once they do buy a car, blacks and Latinos alike are often required to pay a significantly higher annual percentage rate than whites on car loans—on average, 7.5 percent as compared with 6 percent, which amounts to a difference of $900 over the life of a six-year loan on a $20,000 car.[15] Car insurance differentials, while they vary from state to state, are even more striking. In California, a recent proposal to eliminate zip code insurance premium pricing by the California Insurance Commission (the outcome of which has yet to be resolved) illuminates the problem. The Consumers Union found that California's largest insurance companies typically charge a female driver with a perfect driving record and twenty-two years driving experience an average of 12.9 percent, or $152, more if she lives in a predominantly Latino zip code versus a non-Hispanic white area. In some cases, differentials were as high as 66 percent—the surcharge imposed on the predominantly African American residents of Baldwin Hills, California.[16]

Another less well documented, but perhaps more formidable barrier to car ownership among black urbanites is the lack of affordable parking in many of their neighborhoods. Suburban development around cities such as New Orleans was designed with car ownership (as well as white flight) in mind, but the older housing stock and apartment buildings that dominate many urban areas do not include garages or space set aside for parking. Moreover, as tourism and business travel increasingly displace other forms of commerce in many historic cities, even less parking is available to residents—making car ownership ever more expensive and difficult in many inner-city neighborhoods.[17]

Personal Responsibility? The Racial Politics of Evacuation

Given the systemic racial discrimination of automobile sales and maintenance, it is little wonder that so many African Americans in pre-Katrina New Orleans had no access to a car. But when the disaster struck, the carless paid a high price for being black. Evacuation plans that the city of New Orleans and the state of Louisiana had in place before the storm generally worked well for those with access to vehicles, as several transportation planners have pointed out. "Travel conditions were good during the evacuation period," observes Todd Litman. Several other planners characterize the evacuation of New Orleans as "the most successful highway based evacuation in U.S. history." One of the major reasons it was "so effective," they observe, was careful planning on the part of city and state officials. In the wake of the "highly criticized evacuation" during Hurricane Ivan in 2004, an "Improved Contraflow Plan" to regulate highway traffic during emergency evacuations had been developed by the state a few months before Katrina. An elaborate diversion of traffic off freeways onto alternative routes successfully cleared the interstate for car-owning evacuees leaving the area that the hurricane was projected to hit.[18]

Left wholly unplanned, however, was the evacuation of what pre-Katrina disaster plans estimated to be 200,000 to 350,000 New Orleans residents who lacked access "to reliable personal transportation." The need to provide an evacuation plan for this population was discussed as early as 2001, in a *Scientific American* article aptly titled "Drowning New Orleans." Written by veteran science reporter, Mark Fiscetti, the article warned, "If a big, slow-moving hurricane crossed the Gulf of Mexico on the right track, it would drive a sea surge that would drown New Orleans under 20 feet of water"—a prediction that was repeatedly reiterated in other broadly circulated publications.[19] Moreover, a July 2004 Federal Emergency Management Agency simulation of a category 3 hurricane on the southern Louisiana coast (about the size of Katrina once it hit land) projected 61,290 dead and 38,257 injured or sick in the wake of a catastrophic flood in New Orleans. Yet, the City of New Orleans Comprehensive Emergency Management Plan addressed this well-documented flaw in its evacuation plans in only the vaguest terms. Its guidelines were (and still are) directed toward car owners. Indeed, both before and long after the hurricane, the city's Web page provided no instructions whatsoever for leaving the city via any other means of transportation. In theory, however, the city promised such instructions would materialize as needed: "special arrangements will be made to evacuate those who are unable to transport themselves or who require specific lifesaving assistance. . . . Additional personnel will be recruited to assist in the evacuation procedure."[20] But as Hurricane Katrina approached, no such arrangements took place.

On the contrary, city, state, and federal officials alike did not organize the deployment of the four hundred school buses and New Orleans Regional Transit buses in daily use for the evacuation of the city, let alone secure the additional one thousand to two thousand buses that would have been required to ferry all the residents who lacked transportation out of the city. Moreover, the transit buses, which are variously estimated as having had the potential to fill between 25 percent and 80 percent of the city's transportation needs if properly used during the disaster, were severely underutilized. Deployed on an ad hoc basis by officials during the emergency, they were used "without a detailed action plan" and for a limited time only.[21] On August 27 and 28, New Orleans Regional Transit buses carried people from ten pickup locations to the emergency relief center at the Superdome. But after Katrina hit, most of the city's buses were parked in municipal lots. Although New Orleans residents were still seeking shelter from the storm, "the city failed to designate buses or drivers for post-landfall evacuations." "Independent creatures of state law," neither the Regional Transit Authority nor the New Orleans Parish School Board report directly to the city, and neither agreed to provide the drivers needed to operate the buses during the evacuation.[22] As a result, many city buses remained stationary long after Katrina passed. Parked in the path of the storm, approximately two hundred school buses were submerged in floodwaters that engulfed the city, the gas and oil that seeped out of their waterlogged engines and fuel tanks adding to the "toxic soup" left by Katrina.[23] Ravaged by water, the stranded buses formed a grim monument to the city's planning failures that local wags nicknamed the "Mayor Ray Nagin Memorial Motor Pool."[24]

With many of the city's municipal and school buses submerged, on September 2 the mayor made a desperate appeal for buses. "I need 500 buses," Nagin announced on a local radio station; "get every doggone Greyhound in the country."[25] Asked nine days later about his failure to utilize city buses to evacuate its residents, Nagin admitted that no plans had ever been made to ensure that the city had bus drivers in place during an evacuation. "Sure, there was a lot of buses out there," he conceded. "But guess what? You can't find drivers that would stay behind with a Category 5 hurricane, you know, pending down on New Orleans. . . . We had the assets, but the drivers just weren't available."[26] Indeed, all available evidence suggests that they were never asked to stay.

Likewise, the New Orleans Harbor Police, whose boats could have been used to rescue those stranded by the high water, were nowhere to be found by September 1, having been ordered to flee the city for higher ground on August 30. Left behind when buses stopped running and the harbor police moved their boats to safer waters were African American families such as the

Thomas family. The Thomases owned one car, a five-seat Chevy Cavalier, but ultimately did not use it, because it could not accommodate their nine-year-old nephew and five children—several of whom were young enough to require car seats. With eight people to evacuate, they faced a dilemma when the hurricane hit. As the waters kept rising, Brian Thomas grew increasingly worried and contemplated tossing the car seats out of his car and piling in the whole family. But with radio reports warning that Louisiana State Police would detain evacuees who traveled in overloaded and unsafe cars, he decided to stay put—a decision he regretted in the wake of the storm when the family ended up spending two scorching and waterless days huddled on their roof.[27] Other occupants of New Orleans's Ninth Ward, where less than 70 percent of the households own cars, had even less choice about staying. Twenty-year-old Javelin Coleman, who was stranded there along with her infant son, left only when the waters were high enough to allow her to commandeer a canoe.[28]

Coleman and others were left unserved by the city of New Orleans, which offered them no transportation out of the city during the evacuation of New Orleans, and still has no plan in place for the much smaller number of evacuees likely to be stranded in the event of further hurricanes on the south Louisiana coast. The city's Comprehensive Emergency Management Plan (which is comprehensive in name only) still offers evacuation guidelines instructing city residents to take "only one vehicle" or "go with a neighbor, friend, or relative . . . if you need a ride"—although events during Katrina have documented that people who do not own cars tend to cluster in the same neighborhood and therefore are likely to have friends and neighbors who also do not own cars. In May 2006, the city updated its Web site with a new "City Assisted Evacuation Plan" (CAEP). Designated as "an evacuation method of last resort," that "is not intended to replace the individual's personal responsibility in planning his or her own evacuation," the CAEP could not speak more eloquently on the continuing perils of traveling black in post-Katrina New Orleans. It links personal responsibility with car ownership and offers limited prospects for actual evacuation to those who do not own a vehicle. Moreover, as of January 2008, the 2006 CAEP remained featured on the City of New Orleans official Web site. It was in the spring of 2007 when the announcement "of a high-tech emergency notification system that will assist in delivering real-time messages in times of emergency" appeared. The notification system will supply emergency information via e-mail and/or cell phone to first responders and other city residents who register for the service. But it offers no new transportation alternatives for carless city residents. According to its still-posted 2006 plan, the city plans to once again use buses to take them to local shelters such as the Convention Center and suggests that arrangements will be made to take evacuees elsewhere, by rail, plane, and bus, and with the aid of Amtrak, the airlines, and the state transportation department.[29]

But when the plan was first announced, the city had not completed arrangements to this effect with Amtrak, the airlines, or the state transportation department—which told CNN in 2006 that while willing to help, "it considered it the city's responsibility to get people out of town." Moreover, as of spring 2007, "the federal government had not given its approval for New Orleans to use the train system in the event of an evacuation," and I could find no evidence that approval had been granted in the following year.[30] Accordingly, with the mayor's Memorial Motor Pool still out of commission, the city has "no more than 100 buses available for the job of moving an estimated 10,000 people, and the bus drivers have not agreed to stay." Indeed, the fundamentals of its current evacuation plan, as estimated by CNN's Gulf Coast bureau, would simply reproduce "a scenario reminiscent of the chaos when Hurricane Katrina hit the city."[31]

At issue here is not just what may happen in New Orleans or elsewhere should the Gulf Coast flood again. Rather, the failure of black mobility in the case of Katrina underscores the continuing racial disparities in access to transportation across the nation. The inability of black people to protect their own bodies because of social barriers reveals that *Plessy* is not just a historical artifact, but an enduring legacy in the United States. Roughly 80 percent of federal and local transportation spending is devoted to highways, with only 20 percent going to public transportation. Like the railways at the turn of the twentieth century, highways today can claim their ground by right of eminent domain.[32] A product of public taxation, public spending, and legal claims to public utility, highways do not serve all Americans equally. Highways connected suburban residents to businesses and thereby helped suburban development. Those same highways also cut through inner-cities and thus contributed to the destruction of urban neighborhoods—where residents often lacked the resources and organizational skills needed to resist such developments.

The United States sustains a transportation culture that has retroactively framed the achievements of Rosa Parks and other civil rights activists who participated in the Montgomery Bus Boycott of 1957 and the Freedom Rides of 1961 as pyrrhic victories. Largely unused by many black urbanites, many of our highways are designed and constructed to serve the transportation needs of white suburbanites. Indeed, just as the development of New Orleans as a nineteenth-century port city took shape around waterways, the development of twentieth-century New Orleans took shape around highways, built to link the city to wetland suburban developments. The ironies of this infrastructural reformation abound. Safer than the lowland population of the center city to begin with, and evacuated in an orderly fashion according to the city's carefully designed Contraflow Evacuation Plan, inhabitants of New Orleans's suburban developments emerged from Katrina largely unscathed, but not simply as a result of their personal responsibility. Rather, their safety was assured because the city took responsibility for providing for them in the event of an emergency, as well as facilitating, at substantial cost, their day-to-day transportation—a responsibility that municipalities such as New Orleans owe to all Americans regardless of race or car ownership.

In practice, ensuring this access to transportation under federalism has been difficult, as Roland Anglin shows in his essay, "The Ship of State." The market and local provisions for emergencies typically create winners and losers in disasters. And among the losers can be public safety as well as public access to transportation—as Karen O'Neill's work underscores. In disasters such as Hurricane Katrina, access to public transportation is matter of public safety; and like New Orleans's waterways, the city's largely black pedestrians were ill-served by a long history of federal and local land-use planning that has favored economic development over social and environmental concerns. The Katrina crisis betrayed the early promise of *Brown v. Board of Education* and of Justice Harlan's dissent in *Plessy v. Ferguson*, which both held out the hope that the government should and would take responsibility for ensuring the freedom of mobility for all its citizens. It is only when such responsibilities are universally honored that all Americans can be said to have achieved the "power of locomotion" envisioned by Justice Harlan.

NOTES

1. Adam Rothman, *Slave Country: American Expansion and the Origins of the Deep South* (Cambridge, Mass.: Harvard University Press, 2005), 83.

2. Roger A. Fischer, "A Pioneer Protest: The New Orleans Street-Car Controversy of 1867," *Journal of Negro History* 53, no. 3 (1968): 219–233.

3. Dale A. Somers, "Black and White in New Orleans: A Study in Urban Race Relations, 1865–1900," *Journal of Southern History* 40, no. 1 (1974): 27.

4. *Plessy v. Ferguson*, 163 U.S. 537 (1896), reprinted in *Documents in American Constitutional and Legal History*, ed. Melvin L. Urofsky and Paul Finkelman (New York: Oxford University Press, 2002), 1:540.

5. *Plessy*, Justice Harlan, dissenting, in ibid.

6. See, for example, Benjamin Kilpatrick, "Katrina and Class: A (Missed) Wake-up Call," Molinari Institute, January 7, 2006, http://praxeology.net/Kilpatrick-Katrina.htm; and C. L. Cole, "Katrina's Wake-up Call," *Journal of Sport and Social Issues* 29, no. 4 (2005): 367–368.

7. Audie Cornish, "Katrina Took Deadly Toll on Elderly," NPR, March 5, 2006, http://www.npr.org/templates/story/story.php?storyId=5242064; Alix Speigel, "Katrina's Impact on Elderly Still Resonates," NPR, March 1, 2006, http://www.npr.org/templates/story/story.php?storyId=5239019.

8. Bob Quigley, "Six Months after Katrina: Who Was Left Behind—Then and Now," Common Dreams.org, http://www.Commondreams.org/views06/0221-36.htm. Quigley draws on Federal Emergency Management Agency (FEMA) statistics.

9. Meizhu Lui, Emma Dixon, and Betsy Leondar-Wright, "Stalling the Dream: Cars, Race, and Hurricane Evacuation," United for a Fair Economy's Third Annual Report, *State of*

the Dream, 2006, http://www.faireconomy.org/files/pdf/stalling_the_dream_2006.pdf. See also Robert D. Bullard and Glenn S. Johnson, *Just Transportation: Dismantling Race and Class Barriers to Mobility* (Stony Creek, Conn.: New Society Publishers, 1997).

10. See, for example, Steven Raphael and Lorien Rice, "Car Ownership, Employment, and Earnings," *Journal of Urban Economics* 52, no. 1 (2002): 109–130; Thomas W. Sanchez, "The Connection between Public Transit and Employment: The Cases of Portland and Atlanta," *Journal of the American Planning Association* 65, no. 3 (1999): 284; William Colman, "Schools, Housing, Jobs, Transportation: Interlocking Metropolitan Problems," *Urban Review* 10, no. 2 (1978): 92–107.

11. Lui et al., "Stalling the Dream."

12. Todd Litman, "Lessons from Katrina: What a Major Disaster Can Teach Transportation Planners," *Victoria Transport Policy Institute* (2005): 5.

13. Marjorie Whigham Desir, "Are You Being Taken for a Ride—African-Americans Charged More for Automobiles," *Black Enterprise*, April 1997.

14. Ian Ayres and Peter Siegelman, "Race and Gender Discrimination in Bargaining for a New Car," *American Economic Review* 85, no. 3 (1995): 307.

15. Consumer Federation of America, "African-Americans Pay Higher Auto Loan Rates but Can Take Steps to Reduce This Expense," February 15, 2006, http://www.consumerfed.org/elements/www.consumerfed.org/file/finance/auto_loan_press_release_5-7-07.pdf.

16. "Regulatory Changes Would Disallow Zip-Code Insurance Rating," http://info.insure.com/car_insurance/zip_code_proposal.html.

17. Scholarly literature on parking and car ownership is hard to find, but cities such as New York and New Orleans typically have "limited and high cost parking," which in the case of New Orleans is not offset by effective public transportation. Robert I. Dunphy and Kimberly Fisher, "Transportation, Congestion, and Density: New Insights," *Transportation Research Record* 1552 (1996): 91. On tourism and the limits of public transportation in New Orleans, see Robert C. Post, "The Machine in the Garden," *Society for the History of Technology* (2006): 91–94. On issues of parking and planning in terms of "new urbanism" and high-density urban renewal, see Philip R. Berke and Thomas J. Campanella, "Planning for Postdisaster Resiliency," *Annals of the American Academy of Political and Social Science* 604 (2006): 192–207.

18. Litman, "Lessons from Katrina," 1; Brian Wolson et al., "Louisiana Highway Evacuation Plan for Hurricane Katrina: Proactive Engagement of a Regional Evacuation," *Journal of Transportation Engineering* (January 2006): 1.

19. Mark Fiscetti, "Drowning New Orleans," *Scientific American* 285, no. 4 (2001): 76–85; Eric Berger, "Keeping Its Head above Water," *Houston Chronicle*, December 1, 2001, http://www.hurricane.lsu.edu/_in_the_news/houston.htm; Joel K. Bourne, "Gone with the Water," *National Geographic*, October 2004, 92, http://www3.nationalgeographic.com.

20. "City of New Orleans Comprehensive Emergency Management Plan," May 2005, http://www.tornadochaser.net/city_of_new_orleans_comprehensive.htm.

21. Litman, "Lessons from Katrina," 12.

22. Senate Report 109-322, "Hurricane Katrina: A Nation Still Unprepared," May 2006, 359, 250, http://www.gpoaccess.gov/serialset/creports/katrinanation.html.

23. "Toxic soup" was a term widely used to describe the floodwaters that covered New Orleans in the summer and fall of 2005, although more recent research suggests that

both these waters and the sediment they left behind were not as hazardous as that term suggests. Jennifer Wilson Fisher, "Health and the Environment after Hurricane Katrina," *Annals of Medicine* 144, no. 2 (2006): 153–156.

24. The term appears in variety of sources, including Deroy Murdock's "Multilayered Failures," National Review Online, September 13, 2005, http://www.nationalreview .com/murdock/murdock200509130839.asp.

25. "Mayor to Feds: 'Get off Your Asses,'" transcript of radio interview with New Orleans's Mayor Nagin, September 2, 2005, http://www.cnn.com/2005/US/09/02/nagin .transcript.

26. Tim Russert interview with Ray Nagin on NBC's *Meet the Press*, September 11, 2005, http://www.msnbc.msn.com/id/9240461.

27. The Thomases' story appears in Will Haygood, "'To Me, It Just Seems like Black People Are Marked,'" *Washington Post*, September 2, 2004.

28. Javelin Coleman's experience is recorded in Marcus Franklin and Jamie Thompson, "Crisis Raises Questions of Race," *Saint Petersburg Times*, September 2, 2005.

29. See http://www.cityofno.com/portal.aspx?portal=98&tabid=1&load=~/CNO/Services/ CAEP/CAEPWizard.ascx.

30. See Chuck Hustmyre, "Hurricane Season 2007: No Shelter in Place," *HS Today*, June 2007, http://www.hstoday.us/content/view/623/92; and "Testimony of Glenn M. Cannon," February 2008, http://transportation.house.gov/Media/File/Rail/20080211/ FEMA%20Testimony.pdf.

31. Susan Roesgen, "New Orleans Evacuation Plan Has Holes," CNN.com, May 22, 2006, http://www.cnn.com/2006/US/05/11/new.orleans.evacuation.index.html?iref= newssearch.

32. Bullard and Johnson, *Just Transportation*.

3

A Slow, Toxic Decline

Dialysis Patients, Technological Failure, and the Unfulfilled Promise of Health in America

KEITH WAILOO

Hurricane Katrina made private illness experiences and health vulnerabilities shockingly public, and nothing more graphically captures this fact than the drama surrounding dialysis patients in the days after the storm. Their commonplace and everyday problems were thrown open to deeper scrutiny, framed as a metaphor for the tragic moment and, as I shall argue, a metaphor for the nation's unfulfilled political and economic commitments. Many commentators rightly connected the story of these patients to the uneven and endemic health vulnerabilities that long predated the storm. "How many of the dead will turn out to be dialysis patients?" asked one expert. One July 2007 study answered that "the best guess is that of over 5,800 Gulf Coast dialysis patients affected by Katrina, 2.5 percent died in the month after the storm—although given the high mortality rate among dialysis patients, it is difficult to determine how many deaths were storm-related."[1] Commentaries placed dialysis squarely in the center of political analysis. In one ironic letter in the *San Diego Union Tribune*, the writer voiced deep disdain for the delayed and incompetent federal response: "And across the ocean in his supposed cave, I can picture Osama bin Laden, who can manage to get dialysis while, on Thursday, Charity Hospital in NO had only fruit punch to offer its patients."[2] In this telling, the story epitomized government's broken promise to its most needy citizens.

This chapter examines what the appearance of dialysis patients in the story of Katrina reveals about race, health, region, and the nation's commitments. In the hours and days following the storm, diabetics and patients whose kidneys had failed and who depended on dialysis technology figured prominently in news coverage. They were unable to move themselves out of harm's way for want of transportation and further immobilized because of their health challenges. "Thousands of victims of Hurricane Katrina face homelessness and devastation," announced the National Kidney Foundation, "but kidney patients without access to dialysis treatment face life-threatening danger."[3] They needed what had become over the previous two decades a standard medical treatment to cleanse their blood, but the instrument itself depended on clean water, running electricity, and medical staff and facilities. Many of these patients were diabetics whose kidneys had failed. Requiring regular dialysis treatments, such people found themselves stranded in airports, in homes, in the Superdome—tethered to a city without electricity and lacking medical services—suffering from a slow, toxic demise as impurities built up in their bodies. This small sub-set of victims symbolized a peculiarly American kind of vulnerability arising from poor access in a technology-rich environment. Among the most vulnera-ble of the vulnerable, they became—along with the elderly in nursing homes, the residents of Charity Hospital, the cancer patients, and other infirm citizens of the region—a graphic symbol of Katrina's toll. One Washington, D.C.–based kidney specialist predicted in the *Washington Post* on September 13, 2005, "It's going to take months, if not years, to actually find out what proportion of the dead were actually dialysis patients."[4]

As one physician in the Tulane University Department of Nephrology later stated, the dialysis machines were part of a more extensive technological system that failed: "I had a group of about seven or eight patients that we needed to take care of, then we got ten additional patients from the Superdome brought by the police, and a few people walked into the ER needing dialysis, . . . [but in the immediate wake of the storm] we didn't have enough water pressure." At first, only two machines could be run, but then "about six or seven hours later we lost the pressure completely."[5] The other problem for such patients was that, even if the pressure returned, the water was not potable. And clean water was also essential for running these machines that do the essential work of the kidneys—removing toxins from the blood that build up slowly in the course of normal life. As another New Orleans specialist later noted, "People didn't understand the extent to which they were a special needs population."[6] In these stranded patients, even those who were evacuated "were very worse off for the trip they had to make under the conditions. . . . People were lined up [for example] waiting for machines up in Baton Rogue."[7]

These people's predicaments were powerful reminders of health promises unfulfilled in America. They were a subset of Louisiana's many health problems, which included low immunization rates; high rates of stroke, diabetes, and heart disease; and deteriorating public health infrastructure.[8] All of these problems had social origins. Susceptibility to kidney failure, for example, had grown over the decades, making the population more and more dependent on dialysis. And since the early 1970s, the federal government had sanctioned a special relation-ship between patients and dialysis through a law granting universal access to the technology. It was, then, a technology with a unique place in the health-care system—a federally mandated entitlement for citizens if their kidneys failed.

Thus the dialysis story in Katrina was not merely a local crisis; it was in some sense a national one. But the federal guarantee of dialysis meant little if water, electricity, equipment, and cooperation in the social delivery of care did not exist.

Dialysis patients turned up as a recurring leitmotif in the media's efforts to convey the gravity of the Katrina story.[9] The failure of dialysis technology—like failed levees, canals, and pumps—revealed the weakness inherent in a technologically reliant society. And just as proximity to the levees and residence in low-lying homes had a distinctly racial cast, so too did the story of dialysis.

The Stroke Belt, the Diabetes Burden, and Dependence on Dialysis

New Orleans and Louisiana are part of the so-called stroke belt—a stretch of states across the American Southeast associated with high rates of stroke and an array of hypertension-related disorders.[10] Since the 1940s, experts have pondered the reasons, speculating that high-fat diets and obesity, smoking, genetic predisposition, or other unknown factors are responsible for these elevated rates.[11] The "belt" remains an enigma, but many experts believe that diet and higher rates of hypertension among African Americans put them at increased risk of stroke. The high rate of hypertension was also linked to other ailments. "In the Southeast," noted one researcher in 1994, "hypertension is the most common cause of ESRD [kidney failure], followed by diabetes mellitus, occurring most frequently in older minority patients, particularly blacks." Kidney failure—the endpoint in a cascade of other ailments—was, he concluded, "a Southern epidemic."[12]

The correlation between end-stage renal disease (ESRD), diabetes, and being black cut in many directions—and these links were also associated with income. Diabetes is believed to be caused by "a complex interplay of genetic, cultural, social and environmental influences, as well as healthcare inequities."[13] In Louisiana as elsewhere, the correlation between poverty and diabetes is also well established. Some 11 percent of black people in the state and 7.2 percent of white people were diabetic in the years before Katrina, among the highest occurrences in the nation. These rates rise in the population as incomes falls, and as a 2004 report noted, nearly 16 percent of people in Louisiana with incomes under $15,000 per year were diabetic. Conversely, the income correlation with diabetes showed that for people with incomes over $50,000 per year, the percentage dropped to 4.8 percent. Only a few months before Katrina, in March 2005, one physician cautioned that given this complex array of factors— from diet to obesity to poverty and diabetes—the vulnerability of black Americans in the region to kidney failure was disturbingly high.[14]

By 2005, Louisiana was second only to Washington, D.C., in the per capita rate of kidney failure, much of which resulted from diabetes. New Orleans was not exactly "ground zero" for American diabetes, but it was a close second—a major player in a national epidemic of kidney disease.[15] But, as one commentator noted a week before Katrina struck, these ailments were not high-profile disorders like AIDS, breast cancer, and prostate cancer—and the regional health challenges, although known to health experts, did not receive sustained or widespread public attention. "Where," he wondered, "are the lapel ribbons and the walkathons [for diabetes]?"[16]

Kidney failure is a less glamorous form of debility—a less prominent force in the identity-based struggles of patients' advocates for public attention and resources. It was this often-concealed, private reality that came starkly into view in the days after Katrina struck, propelling dialysis patients into the public eye as they battled for health services. Media coverage of Katrina—by spotlighting dialysis—made momentarily visible a form of debility, dependence, and death that is widespread and intimately linked to the region's culture and geography. But the sudden appearance of dialysis also draws our attention to a deeper story of a region and the nation: the story of kidney failure and dialysis intersects, as we shall see, with other stories about how technology-based dependence came about in the first place and feeds vulnerability, and how the promise of government and the federal entitlement to health services had brought these sufferers to a new political crossroads.

Who Lives and Who Dies: Vulnerability and Technological Dependence in Historical Perspective

To look more deeply into the story of diabetics and dialysis is to uncover a complex historical relationship between human beings, disease, technology, and the role of government in health care—a history that illuminates the irony of technology in the making of vulnerability. Indeed, this was not the first time dialysis made national headlines. Several decades before Katrina struck, dialysis patients had figured as an important touchstone in the national debate about vulnerability, government, and citizenship.

As the historian Steven Peitzman notes, a profound racial disparity exists in cities across the nation in the rate of kidney failure, which is three or four times higher for blacks than whites.[17] The disproportion, "apparent to all by the 1980s," he writes, has numerous origins, but principal among them is diabetes and less access to early kidney care, leading to organ failure in end-stage renal disease (ESRD). "Whatever the reasons for so much ESRD among blacks in the United States and elsewhere," Peitzman observes, a convergence has emerged between the dialysis experience and the broader African American experience: "'[G]oing on dialysis' is nearly as familiar a part of African-American life in the cities as is going to church."[18]

But there is also a deeper backstory, for type 2 diabetes—in which the body does not produce enough insulin or becomes resistant to insulin—is often linked to diet and obesity. Thus, the economic geography of the region and the history of the southern diet, particularly New Orleans cuisine, also have become implicated in the question of dialysis reliance. The Big Easy, after all, has long been associated with good eating—carrying one set of meanings for tourists and another for residents. So, many people dependent on dialysis in New Orleans were brought to this fateful juncture with Hurricane Katrina through particular historical and social processes; yet their stories cannot be separated from additional social factors that are important in explaining how, and why, peoples' kidneys can fail—from urinary tract infection (severe, untreated) to lead poisoning and HIV. Thus were race, diet, and a host of urban factors, along with poverty, implicated in higher rates of diabetes.

Dialysis in this country—a technology to allay the effects of slow, toxic death—has always been intimately tied to the logic of American government and to the debate over government's relationship to vulnerable citizens. The ability to artificially cleanse the blood of harmful waste products via hemodialysis emerged as a technical possibility after World War II, but access to the lifesaving technology became an entitlement through federal law in the early 1970s—at a crucial moment in U.S. history. With passage of Public Law 92–603 in October 1972, a "dialysis entitlement" within a Social Security amendment committed the nation to paying the cost of dialysis for all patients (wealthy or poor) whose kidneys had failed. These people with end-stage renal disease were beneficiaries of a liberal era of still-expanding government services.[19] The driving force behind the ESRD legislation was the glaring inequalities of the era—with the shocking role played by income and economic privilege in private access to dialysis, thus determining who lived and who died. "In the earliest years of chronic dialysis," observes Steven Peitzman, "the number of people who might benefit from the procedure exceeded its availability."[20] In the 1960s, hospitals with the still-scarce dialysis machines found that it was necessary to choose worthy recipients from among the many who sought to benefit. In a few well-known cases, hospitals with few dialysis facilities formed panels (criticized as "God committees") to decide on the criteria for distributing access to this rare, life-extending commodity. Precisely because the vagaries of class played such a powerful and unfortunate role in who did and did not get dialysis, pressure for equity grew. ESRD legislation thus sought to remedy these flaws, while building on the unprecedented passage only a few years earlier of Medicare, which ensured federal health coverage for the elderly. The argument for covering ESRD at the time was compelling: American technological prowess was well demonstrated. We could, after all, send men to the moon; surely, the nation could ensure access to lifesaving kidney dialysis. But as one of the Senate staffers involved in the legislation later recalled, "ironically, rather than serving as a demonstration or pilot, the ESRD legislation proved to be the last train out of the station for national health insurance. No other group has had a chance to get on board."[21]

For more than the past three decades, then, the story of dialysis and the government's commitment to extending life has been a political one—tied closely to the growth of the national health-care system and its underlying political and economic commitments. But the growth of dialysis has also spawned a large and growing sector of private, commercial dialysis centers, many of them in the South (where diabetes is more prevalent). And as the incidence of ESRD has increased year by year—"growing about 3 percent a year, fueled by the rise of diabetes"—and the number of dialysis patients has expanded, the cost and profit associated with this unique entitlement has grown too, along with the debate over whether the U.S. as a nation could afford to live up to its commitment to care for these patients.[22]

The story of dialysis and diabetes in Katrina is, in some ways, one of the latest chapters in this unfolding political debate over government's priorities, its citizens, and how the state responds to those in need. The disease and its treatment are also part of the story of growing dependence on a technology that is tied to the ideals of a liberal society. Thus, the emergence of dialysis patients into the national spotlight during Katrina was not dramatically new. Long before the storm struck New Orleans, they had been identified as a particularly vulnerable group, warranting special protection and safeguards. Only a year earlier, New Orleans's Mayor Ray Nagin had acknowledged as much. Looking out into the Gulf at the looming threat of Hurricane Ivan, he observed that the city's "priorities are first to secure the ongoing treatment of seriously ill patients in hospitals and for people on dialysis machines."[23] From the era of the "God committees" into the age of ESRD and Katrina, the history of dialysis showed how society wavers in its commitment to these citizens.[24] Against this political backdrop, it should not surprise us that the plight of dialysis/diabetes patients was one prominent story within the broader Katrina narrative and that it carried powerful technological and historical resonance. These resonances hung in the air as one Florida medic commented when the waters remained high, "people have been without medicine and in some cases without dialysis for coming up on a week," and he reminded listeners about the deadly consequences of the buildup of toxins in the blood if these conditions were to continue.[25]

Dialysis patients were not the only ones made vulnerable by disability, of course; the health effects were widespread, yet technologically dependent dialysis patients often epitomized the crisis. The chairman of the Touro Infirmary Hospital, Stephen Kupperman, observed on September 3 that "the government was totally unprepared for something of this size. . . . We could not get any assistance . . . at first." The hospital ultimately turned to private buses and private air ambulances, with a little assistance from government helicopters, to evacuate patients and staff.[26] Many hospitalized patients could not be moved at all, notes one subsequent study, because "for patients who were disoriented or on respirators on in traction, for example, evacuation posed enormous logistical challenges."[27] But in the news coverage, the diabetics and dialysis patients often stood out. As one New Orleans citizen wrote at the time, "On Tuesday evening, my skeletal neighbor Kip, a kidney-transplant patient, waded home alone by flashlight from the convention center, where there were neither dialysis machines nor buses to get him to one. His last treatment had been four days earlier, and he was bloating. We had to get him out."[28] Another article early in the aftermath reported that a nurse at the United Medical Rehab Hospital in the city worried that "several diabetic patients had been without dialysis for nearly a week" and "after the fruit cocktail and peanut butter ran out, the staff broke into the candy and drink machines for sugary items to keep patients from going into shock."[29] Her voice cracking, she complained, "these are people who are not going to make it." Reports on September 5 from a hospital in Atlanta found that of those who fled, "many survivors are shell-shocked, unable to eat or sleep. Some need intravenous hydration; others suffer from not receiving regular dialysis treatment."[30] And nine days later, the *Wall Street Journal* bemoaned that "health officials are searching for hundreds of dialysis patients"—about half of the 3,000 or 3,500 patients whose dialysis centers were destroyed were unaccounted for.[31] And a year later, dialysis continued to frame the storm's effects. One reassessment of life and death at the Houston Astrodome (where many New Orleans residents had been taken) commented that "doctors, administrators and staff from the Harris County Hospital District created a 'virtual hospital without beds' at the Astrodome. Among the seventeen thousand cases handled at the clinic were kidney patients in desperate need of dialysis and diabetics suffering from lack of insulin."[32]

Coverage of the human drama of patients dying while waiting for dialysis inevitably blurred the more complex issues of region, class, race, technology, history, disease, and government that had created this crisis. The story of dialysis provoked some to see New Orleans as a city outside the narrative of American technological progress, a city left behind. For some observers, dialysis became a vehicle for talking about profound failures to progress. In the midst of the wreckage, one observer described a "frail fellow, a diabetic whose limbs are too swollen to walk . . . unable to obtain dialysis treatment for a week, being pushed along in a wheelchair by an elderly friend."[33] Seeing the sad picture, one disgusted resident spat out, "We are a third world city in a first world country."[34] Frequently using the word "primitive," CNN's Sanjay Gupta reported from the airport that "the utter lack of coordination" combined with the devastating impact of the water throughout the city meant that "it was more primitive than what we saw in Iraq. In some ways, it was more primitive than what we saw in Sri Lanka during the tsunami as well."[35] And reflecting on the story of dialysis patients, another Tulane-based nephrologist recalled, "conditions were pretty primitive for the period of time from Monday when the storm hit until Friday when the complete evacuation went on."[36]

Understanding diabetes and dialysis (with its unique national history and regional profile) considerably expands our understanding of the failure that was Katrina. The notion that a privileged society with its complex systems of technological care had so obviously failed its most defenseless citizens provoked outrage at the time. But as we now approach the fifth anniversary of the 2005 storm, the story of dialysis and Katrina has largely subsided from the headlines, reemerging from time to time in subtle ways. It is now mostly left to specialists in health and nephrology to ask crucial questions. Where have the dialysis patients of New Orleans gone? How many have died? Will the survivors return? Will the dialysis centers of the city be rebuilt? These questions are, even now, unanswerable because of the massive dispersion of population. Nearly a year after the story, one physician at Tulane noted, "Prior to Hurricane Katrina there were about eight thousand [dialysis] patients in the state of Louisiana. About four thousand of those . . . resided in the New Orleans metropolitan area. . . . And since the storm I think it's only half the level."[37] Another Tulane physician noted that two of the three university dialysis units were not functioning: "Both of those flooded; neither is open right now. One . . . received such structural damage that it will have to be rebuilt." Would it be rebuilt? "You can't open a dialysis unit in a way unless you have patients, and the patients can't come back unless there is a dialysis unit. . . . You can't do one without the other."[38] And a study done two years after Katrina found that "before the 2005 hurricane season, there were 2,011 and 362 dialysis patients residing in the [two] parishes (the Louisiana equivalent to counties) most affected by hurricanes Katrina and Rita, respectively. Each of these parishes had experienced increases in dialysis patient populations over the past 5 years. However, following the storms, there were 1,014 and 316 dialysis patients residing in the affected parishes."[39] Where those patients went remains something of a public health mystery.

The questions embedded in the story of dialysis are microcosms of a large question about the nation's commitment to its people most at risk. In the storm itself, health policy researchers Bradford Gray and Kathy Hebert noted, "the situation was particularly urgent for hospitals that lost power, communications, and water/sewer service, and that couldn't re-supply such essentials as drugs, blood, linen, and food."[40] Many dialysis centers and diabetes care clinics, hard hit that month, disappeared in the months after the storm.[41] "According to figures assembled by the Louisiana Hospital Association (LHA) during the storm," Gray and Hebert continued, "1,749 patients occupied the 11 hospitals surrounded by the floodwaters."[42] In this context, what happened to dialysis patients became a microcosm of the broader social drama. Their dispersion from New Orleans still raises fundamental questions about what kind of new city will emerge in the wake of the storm and whether its medical infrastructure will ever be the same. In the end, the story of the dialysis patients reveals particular faces in the human geography of vulnerability and suffering. But in its broadest features, the story remains a tale about the limits of American technological capacity; the intersecting economic, cultural, and historical dynamics of disease; the changing nature of the government's fragile promises to its vulnerable citizens; and the nation's inability to maintain a steady spotlight on, let alone care for, its people in need.

NOTES

1. "Kidney Specialists Review Plans for Disaster Response," *Science Daily*, June 22, 2007, http://www.sciencedaily.com/releases/2007/06/070620121247.htm. The report summarizes a new finding published in the *Clinical Journal of the American Society of Nephropology*.

2. Lynn Macey, "Letters to the Editor: Hurricane Katrina," *San Diego Union Tribune*, September 7, 2005, B9.

3. "National Kidney Foundation Offers Information, Resources to Kidney Patients Affected by Hurricane Katrina," *PR Newswire*, September 2, 2005, http://www.highbeam .com/doc/1P2-13202169.htm.

4. January W. Payne, "At Risk before the Storm Struck: Prior Health Disparities Due to Race, Poverty Multiply Death, Disease," *Washington Post*, September 13, 2005.

5. Vecihi Batuman (Department of Nephrology, Tulane University Medical Center), interviewed by Richard Mizelle Jr. (graduate assistant, Rutgers University), July 20, 2006.

6. Paul Muntner (Department of Epidemiology, Tulane University Medical Center), interviewed by Richard Mizelle Jr. (graduate assistant, Rutgers University), July 20, 2006.

7. Ibid.

8. National Center for Health Statistics (NCHS), *Health, United States, 2004—with Chartbook on the Trends in Health of Americans* (Hyattsville, Md.: NCHS, 2004), http://www .ncbi.nlm.gov/books/bookres.fcgi/healthus04/healthus04.pdf. Cited in Bailus Walker and Rueben Warren, "Katrina Perspectives," *Journal of Health Care for the Poor and Underserved* 18 (2007): 233–240.

9. An earlier book of mine, *Dying in the City of the Blues* (Chapel Hill: University of North Carolina Press, 2001), provided the starting point for my analysis. In the story of one disease—sickle cell anemia—one can see the intersection of disease, race, and politics in the South, and the ways that we can use the study of particular maladies, pains, and health experiences offers a lens on a broader discourse of race, health, and American society.

10. David Warnock et al., "Prevalence of Chronic Kidney Disease and Anemia among Participants in the Reasons for Geographic and Racial Differences in Stroke (REGARDS) Cohort Study: Baseline Results," *Kidney International* 68 (2005): 1427–1431.

11. Douglas J. Lanska and Lewis H. Kuller, "The Geography of Stroke Mortality in the United States and the Concept of a Stroke Belt," *Stroke* 26 (1995): 1145–1149;

Daniel T. Lackland and Michael A. Moore, "Hypertension-Related Mortality and Morbidity in the Southeast," *Southern Medical Journal* 90 (February 1997): 191–198.

12. Michael A. Moore, "End-Stage Renal Disease: A Southern Epidemic," *Southern Medical Journal* 87 (October 1994): 1013–1017.

13. Janice P. Lea and Susanne B. Nicholas, "Diabetes Mellitus and Hypertension: Key Risk Factors for Kidney Disease," *Journal of the American Medical Association* 94 (suppl.) (August 2002): 7S-15S, quote on 7S.

14. Moore, "End-Stage Renal Disease."

15. There are more than four hundred thousand people on dialysis nationwide. A disproportionate percentage of dialysis centers and patients are in the South.

16. Ranit Mishori, "A Dubious Distinction: The District Is at the Front of a National Surge in Kidney Disease," *Washington Post*, August 23, 2005, F1.

17. Steven J. Peitzman, *Dropsy, Dialysis, Transplant: A Short History of Failing Kidneys* (Baltimore: Johns Hopkins University Press, 2007), 128.

18. Ibid., 129.

19. Richard Rettig, "Origins of the Medicare Kidney Disease Entitlement: The Social Security Amendments of 1972," in *Biomedical Politics*, ed. Kathi E. Hanna (Washington, D.C.: Institute of Medicine and National Academy Press, 1982).

20. Peitzman, *Dropsy, Dialysis, Transplant*, 112.

21. James Mongan quoted in Charles Plante, "Reflections on the Passage of the End-Stage Renal Disease Medicare Program," *American Journal of Kidney Disease* 35 (2000): 48. For a broader discussion of Medicare politics and the place of kidney dialysis within it, see Jonathan Oberlander, *The Political Life of Medicare* (Chicago: University of Chicago Press, 2003).

22. Andrew Pollack, "The Dialysis Business: Fair Treatment?" *New York Times*, September 16, 2007, 1.

23. Nagin quoted in "New Orleans Battens Down Hatches for Hurricane Ivan," *Irish Times*, September 15, 2004, 15.

24. David Sanders and Jesse Durkheimer, "Medical Advance and Legal Lag: Hemodialysis and Kidney Transplantation," *UCLA Law Review* 15 (1968): 357–413; see also Committee on Chronic Kidney Disease, *Report of the Committee on Chronic Kidney Dialysis* (Washington, D.C.: U.S. Bureau of the Budget, 1967); and Rettig, "Origins of the Medicare Kidney Disease Entitlement."

25. M.A.J. McKenna, "Katrina Aftermath: Medical: CDC Flies in to Deal with Health Crisis," *Atlanta Journal-Constitution*, September 4, 2005, 5A.

26. Quoted in Felicity Barringer and Donald McNeil Jr., "Grim Triage for Ailing and Dying at a Makeshift Airport Hospital," *New York Times*, September 3, 2005, A4.

27. Bradford Gray and Kathy Hebert, "Hospitals in Hurricane Katrina: Challenges Facing Custodial Institutions in a Disaster," *Journal of Health Care for the Poor and Underserved* 18 (2007): 283, 298, quote on 286.

28. Quoted in James Nolan, "Our Hell in High Water," *Washington Post*, September 4, 2005, B1.

29. Quoted in Allen G. Breed, "Katrina Survivors Face Tragedy, Triumph," Associated Press Online, August 31, 2005, http://www.ewoss.com/articles/D8CBE5182.aspx.

30. Patricia Guthrie, "Metro Facilities Face Long-Term Health Burden," *Atlanta Journal-Constitution*, September 5, 2005, 1A.

31. Michael J. McCarthy, "The Katrina Cleanup: Health Officials Seek Missing Dialysis Patients," *Wall Street Journal*, September 14, 2005, A10; "Hurricane: Health Officials Search for Missing Dialysis Patients," *American Health Line*, September 14, 2005.

32. Allan Turner, "Katrina: One Year Later," *Houston Chronicle*, August 28, 2006, A1.

33. Rosie DiManno, "Tales of Woe Shame a Nation," *Toronto Star*, September 2, 2005, A1.

34. Quoted in ibid.

35. Tom Foreman, Adora Udoji, Sanjay Gupta, Jamie McIntyre, Jeff Koinange, Barbara Starr, Miles O'Brien, and Soledad O'Brien, "Hurricane Katrina's Aftermath," *American Morning: CNN* (transcript), September 3, 2005.

36. Lee Hamm (nephrologist, chair of the Department of Medical Education, Tulane University), interviewed by Richard Mizelle Jr. (graduate assistant, Rutgers University), July 20, 2006.

37. Myra Kleinpeter (Department of Medicine, Tulane University), interviewed by Richard Mizelle Jr. (graduate assistant, Rutgers University), July 20, 2006.

38. Hamm, interview.

39. M[yra] A. Kleinpeter, "Shifts in Dialysis Patients from Natural Disasters in 2005," *Hemodialysis International* 11, suppl. 3 (October 2007): 33. As another study by a Baton Rouge nephrologist notes, "No matter how quickly a dialysis unit may reopen after some local or regional disaster, there exists the real possibility that the facility may experience economic consequences that may threaten the very survival of the unit." These challenges include loss of patients and staff, problems in obtaining property or flood insurance, replacement of destroyed dialysis machines, and difficulties in receiving government assistance such as Small Business Administration loans. Robert J. Kenney, "Emergency Preparedness Concepts for Dialysis Facilities: Reawakening after Hurricane Katrina," *Clinical Journal of the American Society of Nephrology* 2 (2007): 812–813.

40. Gray and Hebert, "Hospitals in Hurricane Katrina."

41. Adrienne Allen, Wayne Harris, and Kathleen Kennedy, "A Diabetes Pharmaceutical Care Clinic in an Underserved Community," *Journal of Health Care for the Poor and Underserved* 18 (2007): 255–261.

42. Gray and Hebert, "Hospitals in Hurricane Katrina," 284.

4

The Ship of State

Framing an Understanding of Federalism and the Perfect Disaster

ROLAND ANGLIN

The first images from New Orleans of African Americans stranded on highway overpasses and rooftops waiting to be rescued, and of black bodies decaying in filthy water below them, suggested that historic and structural racism had produced vulnerability by devaluing lives and devaluing a city. This initial story, discussed in detail in this part of the book, also suggested that Hurricane Katrina could happen in other places in America where structural racism has produced similar inequitable settlement patterns. But media images correlating race, class, and vulnerability could not, by themselves, reveal why government institutions that have no obvious relationship to race made these horrors possible. This chapter weaves the problem of race and structural racism into a broader discussion of federalism, arguing that the incrementalism that is characteristic of federalism in the United States produced inaction and confusion at all levels of government during and after Hurricane Katrina. As other chapters in this section of the book demonstrate, incrementalism, as applied to policies on infrastructure, economic development, health, and transportation, meant that some suffered horrifically because they were unable to evacuate or to receive prompt aid, and that many have been unable to recover economically since then.

The hallmarks of American federalism are (1) multiple jurisdictions with overlapping authority and control and (2) incremental policymaking. Policymaking is often driven by limited information, scarce resources, and self-interest on the part of organizations and individuals inside and outside the government who are pressing for or against policy change. The system is not set up to manage long-term ecological and social challenges. Keith Wailoo's chapter on dialysis patients in the wake of Hurricane Katrina provides a pointed example of this, showing how some diseases have been singled out for incremental policies, rather than being addressed in a comprehensive national health policy. In this case, dialysis received exceptionally generous funding from the federal government because the prospect of poor patients dying for lack of government-guaranteed treatment became politically defined as unacceptable.

While the preceding chapters in this section describe how long-term environmental and transportation policies, among others, created a range of social inequalities and how those inequalities have made some populations more susceptible to a disaster, the examination of federalism, herein, argues/ demonstrates that even competent and nonracist officials could not, and perhaps cannot, compensate for the effects of large-scale social problems like inequality, poverty, and segregation. Our government, in part owing to the structural attributes of federalism, cannot respond quickly and effectively to the vulnerabilities that inequality, poverty, and social isolation have created, and which William Rodgers outlines in his later chapter. Viewing vulnerability in this light forces us to reexamine our thinking about what government can and cannot do to protect the American public.

Forensic analyses characterize Katrina as a "perfect disaster." As the Senate Committee on Homeland Security and Governmental Affairs observes in *Hurricane Katrina: A Nation Still Unprepared*,

> the suffering that continued in the days and weeks after the storm passed did not happen in a vacuum; instead, it continued longer than it should have because of—and was in some cases exacerbated by—the failure of government at all levels to plan, prepare for, and respond aggressively to the storm. These failures were not just conspicuous; they were pervasive. Among the many factors that contributed to these failures, the Committee found that there were four overarching ones:
>
> 1. Long-term warnings went unheeded and government officials neglected their duties to prepare for a forewarned catastrophe;
> 2. Government officials took insufficient actions or made poor decisions in the days immediately before and after landfall;
> 3. Systems on which officials relied to support their response efforts failed; and
> 4. Government officials at all levels failed to provide effective leadership.
>
> These individual failures, moreover, occurred against a backdrop of failure, over time, to develop the capacity for a coordinated, national response to a truly catastrophic event, whether caused by nature or man-made.[1]

Failures occurred along the fault lines of the federal system. Indeed, I would argue that the system was designed to be flexible and to disperse duties across many government agencies, and it performed accordingly.

This Senate report fixes on nonstructural variables that policymakers might manipulate: lack of planning, inability to heed warnings, and lack of leadership. In the vein of positive governance typically emphasized in such committee reports, the conclusion is to repair these variables so that preparedness and capacity can be achieved. But what if they cannot be manipulated? What if disaster preparedness (the central question here) is not possible within the existing structure of American governance, which produced very predictable outcomes based on the separation of powers? Asking the question this way opens the discussion to a different set of variables not easily understood or, perhaps more important, not easily changed. In the next section, I revisit the grounding principles of American federalism and link them to disaster management in light of the failures during and after the 2005 hurricanes.

Federalism and Uneven Governance

American federalism is a framework for sharing power among the federal, state, and local governments.[2] Nineteenth-century political debates about federalism began and ended with the Constitution.[3] In the constitutional framework, states cede power and authority to the central government. In a minimalist interpretation of the Constitution, the federal government's role is to take on duties that states cannot or should not perform individually, such as providing for national security, conducting foreign affairs, and promoting free and open markets. State and local governments are responsible for civil defense and threats to public safety. Katrina pointed up tensions between these federal and state powers. Federal statutes, by and large, support the intent that the federal government should respect state government sovereignty, especially regarding police powers. The president, for example, cannot send troops to a state in times of disaster or other crisis unless the governor or state legislature formally requests federal intervention.[4]

Cautious interpretations of the Constitution became less relevant in politics once the federal government undertook the post–Civil War Reconstruction of the South and New Deal interventions into the economy in response to the Great Depression. In the twentieth century, scholars came to view federalism as the legal and conceptual framework that continually creates and resolves conflicts in a country fraught with sectional and cultural differences. Federalism is also seen as the administrative structure of a growing fiscal and regulatory state, which manages both internal challenges (conflict and competition among jurisdictions and constituencies) and problems generated by market failure, changes in civil society, foreign relations, and, now, globalization. Political conflicts and legal disputes that built the regulatory state have allowed states to innovate. They have also created arenas of mutual influence among the federal,

state, and local levels of government, reinforcing the original intent of federalism as an instrument of national democracy.[5]

The logic of federalism has undergone significant transformation in recent
decades.[6] Some students of American government observe that from World
War II until the middle 1970s, the federal government and sublevels of government mainly cooperated. The upheavals brought by the civil rights movement,
the environmental movement, and unchecked inflation in the 1970s saw the
federal government assert new forms of control and coercive action over specific
elements of civil life through intergovernmental grants (incentive federalism)
and regulation.[7] During and after the Reagan administration, federal statutes
and programs devolved responsibility and power over some economic and social
policies to the states and local governments.[8] This was motivated in part by state
and local officials objecting to their perceived loss of authority and protesting
"unfunded mandates," that is, regulations that required state or local action
without providing federal aid to fulfill those duties. Whatever the character of
federalism at any particular time, the underlying dynamic remains the same: the
role of each level of government remains relatively undefined, and responsibility is often a source of intergovernmental conflict and negotiation.

Because the division of powers and funding is produced through contention rather than through top-down fiat, many areas of policy have overlapping, confusing, and contentious lines of authority that may reveal themselves
in times of crisis. Under normal conditions these issues are often debated and
resolved in the courts, but laborious legal battles do not suit crisis decision
making. To return to the example mentioned above, states retain most police
powers, but because the federal government has expanded its disaster "coordination" duties over the years, it is often unclear who should do what during an
emergency that overwhelms local and state authorities. In this dynamic federal
system, it should not surprise us that residents and even state and local officials
expected immediate and heroic federal aid after Hurricane Katrina, even while
federal officials were making public statements that the state and local governments should lead evacuation and relief aid.

Federalism and Disaster Planning and Management

As a result of this political history, disaster management and response remain
very fluid categories in American governance. In 1803, in what is widely seen as
the first instance of federal intervention in a disaster scenario, Congress
approved the use of federal resources to assist the recovery of Portsmouth, New
Hampshire, following a devastating urban fire. Between 1803 and 1950, the federal government intervened in more than one hundred incidents (earthquakes,
fires, floods, and tornados), making federal resources available to affected jurisdictions. These interventions were limited and were delivered in an ad hoc

manner without an established federal role or coordinated response plan. But such aid bills were cited by New Dealers to justify federal aid in response to the economic "disaster" of the Great Depression as well as to natural disasters.[9] For example, Congress gave the Bureau of Public Roads the authority to provide ongoing assistance to states to repair infrastructure damaged by disasters. As Karen O'Neill notes in her chapter, Congress also charged the Army Corps of Engineers with the task of mitigating flood-related threats. But disaster mitigation and relief of all types evolved in piecemeal fashion, often responding to individual events.

The first comprehensive legislation directing federal disaster relief was the Civil Defense Act of 1950. In 1952, President Harry Truman issued Executive Order 10427, which emphasized that federal disaster assistance supplements, rather than supplants, the capacity and resources of state and local governments. This intent was reaffirmed two decades later in President Richard Nixon's 1973 report, "New Approaches to Federal Disaster Preparedness and Assistance." The report stated that "Federal disaster assistance is intended to supplement individual, local, and state resources."[10]

Currently, legislation for providing federal aid in disaster relief, the 1988 Stafford Act, reinforces the principle that response efforts should first utilize state and local resources, establishing a process by which governors may request assistance from the federal government when a disaster overwhelms state and local resources. The act authorizes the president (1) to coordinate all appropriate federal agencies to bring assistance; (2) to issue major disaster or emergency declarations; and (3) to appoint a federal coordinating officer (FCO) to organize the administration of federal relief to local governments and victims of disaster. It created the Interagency Task Force to coordinate the state mitigation programs, chaired by the director of the Federal Emergency Management Agency (FEMA), with relevant federal agencies, state and local government organizations, and the American Red Cross as members.[11]

The Stafford Act also authorizes the president to develop disaster prevention and management programs, to direct federal agencies to provide technical assistance to states, and to distribute grants to develop, update, and improve state disaster management plans.[12] The act mandates creating multihazard maps in cooperation with state and local governments, but these maps are advisory only and carry no real fiscal strictures or directives that prevent development in hazard-prone areas. States are given incentives to develop an approved hazard mitigation plan, but ultimately it is up to the states to determine policy.[13] Local plans must outline the processes for identifying the natural hazards and must describe actions and implementation plans for mitigating them.[14] The Stafford Act is, therefore, an imperfect product of the American system of governance: it sets out only minimal machinery for coordinating work across government levels.

Turning Around the Ship of State

The terrorist attacks on United States cities on September 11, 2001, sparked another crisis for federalism. In response, federal officials linked disaster management and mitigation to security policy by reframing terrorist attacks as another type of disaster and by instructing that disasters of all types be handled by the same set of agencies. This was coupled with new measures, such as grant programs, to encourage states to adopt the new focus on terrorism, technological disasters, and natural disasters as security threats. The resulting policy, set forth in the *National Strategy for Homeland Security*, issued in July 2002 by President George W. Bush, called for a national system for "incident management." The policy integrates many different federal response plans into a single, comprehensive incident management plan covering the gamut of possible emergencies, with the newly created Department of Homeland Security as the umbrella agency overseeing FEMA as well as domestic security agencies.[15]

A wealth of resources were poured into coordination across levels of government. President Bush issued Homeland Security Presidential Directive 5 (HSPD-5) in February 2003. That directive established national homeland security policies, priorities, and guidelines by directing

> the Secretary of Homeland Security to: (a) create a comprehensive National Incident Management System (NIMS) to provide a consistent nationwide approach for Federal, State, and local governments to work effectively together to prepare for, respond to, and recover from domestic incidents, regardless of cause, size, or complexity and; (b) develop and administer an integrated National Response Plan (NRP), using the NIMS, to provide the structure and mechanisms for national level policy and operational direction for federal support to state and local incident managers.[16]

The new homeland security template directed the heads of all federal departments and agencies to adopt the NIMS framework for homeland security activities and to participate in the NRP.

The National Response Plan requires senior officials from all levels of government to work together in order to manage incidents from a single location to "establish a common set of objectives and a single incident plan." Called the Unified Command, officials provide and implement joint decisions on objectives, strategies, plans, priorities, and public communications relating to the incident. As forward-thinking and mindful of planning as this effort is, there are no specific triggers for the National Response Plan. The president's directive, HSPD-5, instructs the secretary of Homeland Security to coordinate the federal government to respond to or recover from terrorist attacks, major disasters, or other emergencies using the following criteria:

- A federal department or agency acting under its own authority has requested the assistance of the Secretary;
- The resources of state and local authorities are overwhelmed and federal assistance has been requested by the appropriate State and local authorities;
- More than one federal department or agency has become substantially involved in responding to the incident; or
- the Secretary has been directed to assume responsibility for managing the domestic incident by the President.[17]

It is of course one thing to call for unity and coordination across state and federal governments and another to administer this idea—and several issues of federalism clouded the question of coordination after Katrina. It is not clear whether the presence of one or more of the stated criteria is enough for a so-called Incident of National Significance (INS) to exist, or if other considerations come into play. Additionally, the NRP does not provide clear direction as to whether the secretary must formally declare an INS or, alternatively, whether an INS is triggered when one or more of these criteria are in place, "including when the President declares a disaster or emergency under the Stafford Act." As *The Federal Response to Hurricane Katrina: Lesson Learned*, a White House report, concludes, "With respect to Hurricane Katrina, when the Secretary of Homeland Security formally declared the event to be an INS on Tuesday, August 30, 2005, arguably an INS already existed, because two of the four HSPD-5 criteria . . . had already been satisfied."[18]

Even if the triggering of an INS had not been at issue, the NRP does not specify clear responses for incidents. In other words, though a great deal of effort has been placed on coordination, the question of a strategic response remains open. During a hurricane, do you evacuate, and how is that done? How do you put in place the assets needed to accomplish a full evacuation? Who makes that call, the mayor, the governor? To exacerbate things, no INS had ever been declared prior to Tuesday, August 30, 2005. Hurricane Katrina was the test case, and the result was evident.

The provisions of the Stafford Act and of the INS, then, follow the pattern of episodic policymaking so characteristic of the history of federalism in the United States: allowing roles to be defined in the course of a specific emergency. Given the historical emphasis on local governments responding first to disasters, provisions for interagency coordination in the Stafford Act and in the INS in themselves do little to clarify which level of government should lead disaster response under which conditions. The political and professional abilities of state and local agencies to motivate coordinated action and to spur federal response are therefore critical for making this system work. The City of New Orleans was singularly unequipped to initiate action within this system.

Considered in this light, assertions by some commentators that the tragedy after the disaster was attributable to the incompetence of specific leaders or specific agencies are not the full story. The American federal system of government has struggled to define strategies for disaster management through decades of trial and error. Layer on this process the questions of who does what, where, and when, and how those duties should be determined politically. Who pays for the significant level of coordination and planning necessary to get the numerous state and local partners to buy into the process, and how do planners build a disaster management infrastructure that can respond well to the next incident, which may occur anywhere at any time? To attempt to plan well for all likely disasters would call into play resources that, as a nation, we are unwilling to spend up front. Such a plan may also require severe limitations on our civil liberties (in the case of preventing terrorism) and on where we choose to work and live (in the case of any of the types of "disasters" as defined by the 2003 National Response Plan). What level or branch of government will take on the politically explosive task of saying to many in the Outer Banks of the Carolinas that they are not allowed to live there because a powerful hurricane might erode the foundations of beachfront property and wash their homes away? Who will tell homeowners in California they that cannot build homes in places where the houses are tinder for fires brought about by long periods of dryness? The answer is that no one will do so, and as a result, the dance between national government and state authority allows our citizens to play multiple games of chance with nature. Governments assign risk, and the public hopes for the best. But the risks inherent in this federalist system are not uniformly distributed; this is a crucial fact that became evident in the wakes of Katrina and Rita. This helps explain why the response to citizens who depended on public transportation as opposed to those who relied on the interstate highway system for private transportation (see Mia Bay's chapter) was so deficient. When calamity does come, the faces of the affected stir us to help, and governments promise to assist in the effort and to rebuild in the aftermath of devastation. But even if they rebuild, the system of governance remains. And the question—can we be protected by government from natural disasters?—persists.

Conclusion

The confused response to the storms by government at all levels should not be chalked up to ineptness and racism at their worst. These are the wrong lenses through which to fully assess the story of Katrina. American government is like a living organism, growing, changing, and attempting to adapt to changing conditions. Like many organic systems, change comes in increments. In the case of government, federalism (and the incrementalism it produces) is a compelling theme that should condition our understanding of what happened in 2005.

Incrementalism is the cornerstone of a federalist-based bureaucracy. Public officials and administrators managing the immediacy of the storms and the aftermath illustrated well the limitations of incrementalism. Agencies at the federal level resisted change when the Department of Homeland Security was created; there was initial confusion about unclear roles and responsibilities. Additionally, during the storm accurate information was scarce, leading to wrong decisions at worst and inaction at best. State and local officials were so overwhelmed that they expected the federal government to provide immediate help on its own initiative, not taking the steps required under federal policy requiring them to first formally request aid from the federal government.

In its basic form, incrementalism provided a ready-made alternative to the model of rational decision making advocated by policy experts after World War II. Managers and organizations, these reformers argued, can rationally anticipate and plan their activities through the identification of a set of decision variables—often sequenced as though they were "if, then" statements used in programming languages. Often termed the "cybernetic model," this approach to decision making promised better outcomes in business and public policy. Others questioned the cybernetic model by pointing out that decision makers, of all stripes, function in an uncertain world characterized by asymmetric information, random events, and a multiplicity of interests that preclude sequenced plans. It is not that planning is impossible but rather that static plans, with all variables and contingences accounted for, are impossible.

By contrast, incrementalism has a much longer history in this country and has broad appeal and applicability. In practice, no public agency, at any level of government, has been capable by itself of changing the fundamental direction of administrative policy from year to year. Policy has been and remains a product of conflict in which administrative and elected officials make decisions designed to comport with their rules and to satisfy their organizational or personal self-interest. Role conflict and battling interests often lead to small changes in policy but also, at times, to paralysis.

Acknowledging the central role of federalism and incrementalism in shaping the effects of Katrina, we might ask, "Will this happen again?" While this question is unanswerable as stated, it is important to note the singular combination of conditions that made the Katrina disaster possible. When the hurricane struck, the government was still in the throes of the 9/11 administrative transformation. This created problems in all jurisdictions hit by the winds and floods of the hurricane, but in New Orleans, the effects were compounded by two related sets of local weaknesses: the City of New Orleans's political system, governing structures, and local economy were poorly organized and underdeveloped, and the city's infrastructure was exquisitely vulnerable physically. As well, it was understandable that local officials expected unusually intensive and prompt federal action, given that the city's basic infrastructure is defined foremost by the federal government's levees, and much of the harm occurred because some of those levees failed. Katrina arrived under the worst conditions and was a unique event. Yet in the context of a prolonged era of reduced public spending and experimentation with devolving authority to states, it is natural for elected officials and administrators at all levels to put off difficult decisions beyond their terms in office, to defer them to another layer of government, or at least to write emergency plans that leave much undefined and underfunded.

NOTES

1. U.S. Senate, Committee on Homeland Security and Governmental Affairs, *Hurricane Katrina: A Nation Still Unprepared* (Washington, D.C.: Government Printing Office, 2006), executive summary, 2; http://www.gpoaccess.gov/serialset/creports/pdf/sr109 -322/execsummary.pdf.

2. One of the earliest systems of American federalism has been termed "dual federalism." In this period, both the state and federal governments were two distinct entities and operated independently of each other.

3. The authority of the central government is one that grew incrementally. The Supreme Court played an important role in creating a stronger central government. Two cases that brought attention and reconciliation to the conflict between the states and the central government are *McCulloch v. Maryland* (1819) and *Gibbons v. Ogden* (1824). It is cases such as these that helped to create a stronger central government.

4. The federal government can intervene and send in troops or other peacekeeping personnel to uphold the U.S. Constitution, as exemplified by President John F. Kennedy's decision to send federal marshals to protect the rights of African American students in Alabama and Arkansas in the 1960s.

5. Samuel H. Beer, "Federalism, Nationalism and Democracy in America," *American Political Science Review* 72 (1978): 9–21.

6. FDR's New Deal ushered in a new wave of federalism, often called "cooperative federalism." This type of federalism was born out of many incremental changes through the courts and the necessity of a national program to pull the nation out from the Great Depression. With the creation and implementation of grant-in-aid programs, local and state governments were offered funding to participate in federal programs. The interplay of local-state-federal governments is identified as one of the hallmarks of cooperative federalism.

7. See Thomas Anton, *American Federalism and Public Policy: How the System Works*, 1st ed. (Philadelphia: Temple University Press, 1989); United States, Advisory Commission on Intergovernmental Relations, *The Condition of Contemporary Federalism: Conflicting Theories and Collapsing Constraints* (Washington, D.C.: Advisory Commission on Intergovernmental Relations, 1981).

8. Another aspect of devolution during the Reagan administration was the contracting out of public works projects to private industries. On the surface, government contracted in size but perhaps not in terms of outlays.

9. Michelle L. Landis, "Fate, Responsibility, and 'Natural' Disaster Relief: Narrating the American Welfare State," *Law and Society Review* 33, no. 2 (1999): 257–318; White House,

The Federal Response to Hurricane Katrina: Lessons Learned, 11, http://www.georgewbush-whitehouse.archives.gov/reports/katrina-lessons-learned.pdf (accessed January 27, 2008).

10. Quoted in National Academy of Public Administration, *Coping with Catastrophe: Building an Emergency Management System to Meet People's Needs in Natural and Manmade Disasters* (Washington, D.C.: National Academy of Public Administration, 1993).

11. White House, *The Federal Response to Hurricane Katrina: Lessons Learned*, 11.

12. The Stafford Act mandates that federal agencies should issue warnings of impending disaster to state and local governments. The president can establish a program providing technical and financial assistance to states and local governments to assist in predisaster planning, and institute cost-effective measures designed to reduce injuries, loss of life, and damage and destruction of property. Federal funds can be provided for technical and financial assistance relating to plans and assessments of community vulnerabilities, with the president's approval. However, states with vulnerabilities must be designated as a natural disaster hazard, and a demonstration of cost-effective public-private partnerships must be made before those funds can be dispersed. Up to 75 percent of costs for mitigation activity (90 percent for impoverished communities) can be covered by the federal funds. An impoverished community is one that consists of three thousand or fewer people that are economically disadvantaged.

13. If the mitigation plan is approved, the federal share can increase up to 20 percent. To receive the increase in funds, the plan must demonstrate eligibility for property acquisition and other mitigation methods, requirements for cost effectiveness, a system of priorities, and a process to assess the effectiveness of a mitigation action.

14. State plans must also identify hazards, risks, and vulnerabilities and put in place multijurisdictional approval and coordination of plan procedures and elements.

15. Officially created in November 2002, the Department of Homeland Security combined some 180,000 employees from portions of twenty-two departments, agencies, and offices of the federal government that touched on some facet of security and disaster management.

16. The National Incident Management System establishes standardized incident management principles and strategies that government, at all levels, and should use to coordinate responses to crises. The central component of the NIMS is the Incident Command System (ICS). The ICS predated the NIMS and has been in development by incident commanders at the federal, state, and local levels. The ICS in theory provides a means to coordinate individual responders and agencies as they respond to an incident. The ICS organization comprises five major functional areas—command, planning, operations, logistics, and finance/administration.

17. White House, *The Federal Response to Hurricane Katrina: Lessons Learned*, 14.

18. Ibid.

PART TWO

Cultural and Psychic Legacies

5

Seeing Katrina's Dead

ANN FABIAN

> For, as every one knows, ghosts of the unburied dead haunt the earth and make themselves exceedingly disagreeable, especially to their undutiful relatives.
>
> —Sir James G. Frazier, "On Certain Burial Customs as Illustrative of the Primitive Theory of the Soul," 1885

I surprise my students sometimes with the idea that a cultural historian looking back on the United States during the first years of the twenty-first century will find a people troubled by unburied bodies—dead bodies and parts of bodies in all the wrong places. For many months, pieces of bodies turned up around the site of the World Trade Center. Construction on the memorial and on new buildings stopped. Just across lower Manhattan, at the South Street Seaport, crowds lined up to see an exhibit featuring the German anatomist Gunther von Hagens's plasticized human bodies. But some visitors wondered about the ethics behind *Body Worlds*. Did each donor sign a consent form? And in Noble, Georgia, the owner of the Tri-State Crematory stopped burning bodies when his furnace broke. In February 2002, Georgia authorities discovered 334 bodies rotting in stacks in outbuildings and moldering in the woods. They charged the owner with three hundred counts of theft by deception. Did the charge of commercial fraud capture what the man had done wrong? During these same years, Native Americans reclaimed and reburied remains of the dead from nineteenth-century museum collections; activists asked for the Vietnamese skulls taken for trophies by U.S. soldiers. Why have these skulls and bones long forgotten become suddenly so visible?[1]

It is clear from these stories that there is something particularly powerful about these misplaced dead. Encounters with dead bodies cut through the surfaces of modern life, exposing something basic and visceral. Anthropologist James Frazier might have included these recent encounters on his long list of meetings between "undutiful relatives" and disagreeable ghosts. But there is also something historically specific about the recent meetings between the living and the unburied and misburied dead. These are the dead bodies of particular times and particular places.

In September 2005, Katrina's dead bodies joined the contemporary parade of ghosts of the unburied. In those first flooded days, we saw bodies on the streets of New Orleans, bodies floating in the receding floodwaters, bodies in Convention Center refrigerators. Rescue workers found bodies in attics, in nursing homes, in piles of rubble, squeezed under moldy couches. Discoveries pushed the coroner's office beyond the breaking point and challenged the death-dealing skills of the people of New Orleans. Over two and a half centuries, residents of that city had grown particularly adept at dealing with the dead. New Orleans boasted architectural wonders to keep the dead above floodwaters, jazz musicians ushering out dead friends, voodoo priestesses who mediated relations between the living and the dead, and vampires who never managed to die. The city's cultural mix had invited a kind of artistry around death; strains of African, African American, Catholic, and Creole ways of doing things were woven together in this city's fragile natural setting.[2]

In those first days after the storm, Katrina's dead were too much even for the artistry of the people of New Orleans. Katrina's bodies stood out as stark reminders of the great vulnerability of these people and this place. The dead were too visible, slipped free from all the cultural nets that help the living deal with the dead. These bodies, it seemed, expressed a failure of the "cultural infrastructure" every bit as glaring as the failures in the city's physical infrastructure. Katrina showed us many things we prefer to keep hidden: our inability to stop hurricanes, of course, but also our neglect of the poverty and racism that made many particularly easy targets of the storm. This failure was obvious to the locals. Patrick McCarthy, a retired electrician, described it this way to a reporter from London, "If you need a metaphor for failure, this is as good as it gets. Everybody should be buried. [This is] an insult to our humanity."[3]

Remembering the exposed bodies, now mostly hidden again, offers a way for us to remember those other hidden wrongs and perhaps to become more dutiful relatives to the people scattered out of New Orleans. Remembering, in other words, can be a forensic exercise, not to learn the identity of the dead or why they died, but a forensic exercise to learn something about those of us who looked at Katrina's dead.

Unexpected Encounters with Corpses

For a few days, it seemed as though dead bodies were everywhere: lying on sidewalks and in puddles of muck, dangling from hedges. Rescue workers found bodies floating along watery streets and bloating in the city's swollen canals, and they complained that corpses, people beyond all help, were making it hard to help survivors. A dead man's shirt tangled itself in a boat propeller, and the search for the living stopped. To make things worse, recently buried bodies came floating out of their new-made graves, as corpses had often done whenever New Orleans had flooded in the past. But this time the confusion was overwhelming, as the summer's dead floated free of their coffins and mixed promiscuously with those killed in the storm. The boundaries around cemeteries, modern cities of the dead, had broken down; the protective levees of a modern logic that was built to separate the living from the dead had failed. "Nothing is where you'd expect it to be," one man said. "Everything is distorted."[4]

Or maybe it was that stories of bodies broke right along with stories of the storm. Reporters knew that the rest of us would sit up and take notice if we saw a body left by the road or a dead woman left in a wheelchair outside the Convention Center. Photographers took pictures of the corpses. And the circulation of the pictures disturbed some of those in charge. The *Los Angeles Times* reported on September 10, 2005, that the Federal Emergency Management Agency (FEMA) planned "to block access to the mass corpse recovery." The scenes would be too "ugly," Lieutenant General Russel Honoré told reporters. "There will be zero access to that operation. You wouldn't want to have pictures of people who are deceased shown in any media. Everybody knows it's a horrific event." Of course, he meant the deaths were horrific, not the pictures of corpses in the media. CNN went to court and got the ban lifted as a violation of the First Amendment. Was the network thinking of the government's prohibition on images of coffins carrying the remains of soldiers killed in Iraq, a ban in effect even as New Orleans flooded? Thanks to the media, we saw pictures of Katrina's dead, though often with identities discretely concealed.[5]

Those of us who had been through the attacks on the World Trade Center and the Pentagon had been schooled in the importance of dead bodies. Even the smallest fragment mattered to mourners who had lost friends and relatives in New York. New Orleans was full of whole bodies, some just rotting in the sun. There were too many pressing concerns for the living to take the time to deal with the dead. The dead would have to wait—wait to be buried or cremated perhaps—but residents and rescue workers in New Orleans performed small gestures over the dead in order to patch their way through a cultural emergency almost as jarring as the physical wreck of the city.

All through the fall of 2005, workers kept discovering bodies in the ravaged city. The body of a woman whose house had been searched three times turned up in the attic. People who returned home discovered dead relatives. The headlines read, "Son Finds Body in Rubble" and "Bodies Still Being Found in Debris." The bodies continued to surface through the next year: "Katrina Victim Found" in May and "Workers Find Body in Flooded Home" in June.[6] These later-discovered remains at least got the care of DNA experts who could figure out who they were, of forensic experts who could figure out why they

died, of a coroner working in a calmer office. But even in the emergency of the
first days, survivors and rescue workers cobbled together rituals for dealing
with the dead; they held makeshift ceremonies over dead bodies and left mark-
ers at places where bodies had been found. They used what they had to try to
put the dead where the dead belonged: blue plastic tarps, black plastic bags,
brown cardboard, red spray paint, and nondenominational prayers.

In those first days, FEMA dispatched its Disaster Mortuary Assistance
Recovery Team (DMORT) to bring in the dead. The DMORT Web site tells you
that the teams are ready for "an incident where more deaths occur than can be
handled by local resources." And then FEMA called in Kenyon International
Emergency Services, a company that earned its stripes handling the dead in the
ruins of the World Trade Center. Quickly, New Orleans had a bureaucratic infrastructure to handle the dead.[7]

DMORT members devised a prayer for the found bodies. "We give thanks
for this person's life. We give thanks that this person was found. We give thanks
for the persons that found them. We ask that they may be made whole in God's
arms and they know peace."[8] While a grammar teacher might have made a few
suggestions, this was surely a prayer written by a committee trying hard not to
offend. It was the right idea—a ritual improvised in a hurry to set the dead apart
from the living, and with thanks for hard-working people performing a difficult
task. It was a ceremony devised to suit the cultural emergency of a natural disaster. DMORT teams were called on not just to collect bodies but also to mourn
the passing of those whose bodies they gathered.

In the first weeks, survivors complained that this bureaucracy actually
failed the dead, although FEMA insisted that DMORT members had been
trained to "treat these remains with dignity" and that they were merely recover-
ing corpses in a methodical and prudent manner. Still, New Orleans Mayor Ray
Nagin complained that FEMA's sluggish response on the body front was disre-
spectful to the deceased. For Senator Mary Landrieu, it was an issue of policy.
The dead must be honored, she said, because "our federal government failed
these individuals in life."[9] Or according to Governor Kathleen Blanco, "In death,
as in life, our people deserve more respect and dignity."[10]

An anthropologist might have anticipated some of the anger, confusion,
and frustration associated with dead bodies, for the proper disposition of the
dead seems to sit at the very heart of what it means to be human. There are
hygienic reasons to bury the dead, of course. But there are cultural reasons just
as pressing. Governor Blanco spoke of what the dead deserved, but she was
speaking for the living. She knew there was something profoundly disturbing in
the signs that a people could no longer bury its dead.

When the literary scholar Robert Pogue Harrison began his recently
published meditation on *The Dominion of the Dead*, he turned first to the

eighteenth-century Italian writer, Giambattista Vico. "To be human means above all to bury," Harrison writes, following one of Vico's peculiar etymologies: "*humanitas* in Latin comes first and properly from *humando*, burying."[11]

Other scholars have shared the sentiment that disposition of the dead with custom and ritual leads straight to what it means to be human. Burial is a basic symbolic act of humanity. In an essay written at the beginning of the twentieth century, just a few years before he would die in the trenches of the First World War, French sociologist Robert Hertz (Emile Durkheim's young student) wrote a study comparing cultural representations of death. "The body of the deceased is not regarded like the carcass of some animal; specific care must be given to it and a correct burial; not merely for reasons of hygiene but out of moral obligation."[12]

These moral obligations lie behind the clumsy but good-hearted prayer composed by the rescue teams in New Orleans. The obligations may be universals, of a sort, but the more interesting questions concern how these universals played out at this particular time and in this particular place: in the United States South, in Louisiana, in New Orleans, in late August and early September 2005, in the commemorative shadows of September 11, 2001, in the early years of an American war in Iraq.

A Double Standard for the Dead

Because Katrina hit New Orleans very close to the fourth anniversary of the terrorist attacks of September 11, 2001, connections between the young century's two riveting tragedies were on many American minds. Some may have paused to remember the incalculable losses from the South Asian tsunami of December 2003, a disaster whose numbers simply dwarfed these American tragedies, but in the United States people linked the two American events and compared the responses.

Here is President George Bush in his radio address on the week following the storm: "This time, the devastation resulted not from the malice of evil men, but from the fury of water and wind."[13] For many in New Orleans, though, there seemed some trace of malice in the slow response and seeming neglect. The floating dead did not expose the malice of evil men, but rather the evil sometimes brought on by thoughtless men. In another context, President Bush fell into an unfortunate phrase; "there was a sense of relaxation at a critical moment," he said. "No one anticipated a breach in the levees."[14]

Pressed to explain this remark, he continued, "When that storm came by, a lot of people said, 'We dodged a bullet.' And that storm came through, people at first said, 'Whew!' There was a sense of relaxation. That is what I was referring to. I myself thought we had dodged a bullet, and you know, because I was listening to people, probably over the airwaves, that a bullet had been dodged. And that is what I was referring to. Of course there were plans in case the levees had been breached. There was a sense of relaxation at a critical moment."[15]

Anger lingered for some who saw a double standard in the treatment of the dead. Contemporary America's inequalities were too much even for death's great leveling powers. Lower Ninth Ward resident Wanda Jackson put it this way to a *New York Times* reporter: "They did not build nothing on 9/11 until they were sure that the damn dust was not human dust; so how you go on and build things in our city?"[16]

Still, what President Bush said was not inaccurate. Many outside the storm area went to sleep thinking that New Orleans had survived. But the floating bodies underlined why his statement felt so wrong. In the weeks following Katrina, searchers found bodies all around the city, but that first visible batch of corpses floated out of zip codes 70117 and 70122, the addresses of the Lower Ninth Ward and Gentilly. It was clear that the city's poverty, and that poverty's particular geography, accounted for many of the bodies. Many of those who died were old and ill, some could not swim, or "perhaps they couldn't drive," said the medical incident commander. One list said six of ten who died were African American. Some tried not to count by race, which after all is a relationship among the living and not the dead, but in contemporary America the impulse to sort, and to sort by race, is unavoidable. It is as important a social fact as the cause of death or the number of dead.[17]

We could make such a list of zip codes, races, and ages for most disasters. But the bodies in New Orleans brought to mind distinctive features of city's cultural history, as well as its geography, ecology, and economy. More than any other American city, New Orleans seems to be a place for the dead. It is true that other cities do have distinct cultures of death—people in Savannah, Georgia, have a way with Gothic tales, and people in Colma, the necropolis just south of San Francisco, boast that the dead outnumber the living—but no city cultivates its dead better than New Orleans, with its jazz funerals, its walking tours of historic cemeteries, and its famous stories of the undead. The city has produced a particular kind of cultural knowledge about death and dead bodies, every bit as characteristic as its food and music. Performance scholar Joseph Roach puts it this way: "Animated by a 'joyful noise,' supported in many instances by the testimony of deep, spirit-world faith, the dead seem to remain more closely present to the living in New Orleans than they do elsewhere—and not only because they are traditionally interred in tombs above ground."

Roach writes about the ways performance preserves cultural memories in a process of substitution he calls "surrogation." "In the life of a community," he writes, "the process of surrogation does not begin or end but continues as actual or perceived vacancies occur in the network of relations that constitutes the social fabric. Into the cavities created by loss through death or other forms of departure, I hypothesize, survivors attempt to fit satisfactory alternates. Because collective memory works selectively, imaginatively, and often perversely, surrogation rarely if ever succeeds. The process requires many trials and at least as many errors."[18] Although Roach describes the process in theoretical language, he captures something of why the floating dead in New Orleans were particularly troubling. The bodies were riveting because for a few days, it looked as though the devastation was so sweeping that even the resourceful people of New Orleans could not incorporate the dead.

Katrina, for a time, broke down the cultural processes of surrogation. The floating dead in New Orleans, the unburied, unidentified bodies, the continuing discovery of corpses suggest that in the wake of Katrina the very process of surrogation, or substitution by which a culture constructs memories out of a past to move into a future, was broken and interrupted. The people of New Orleans, virtuosos of memory and mourning, were stopped in their tracks. If they could not mourn and dispose of the dead, who could? We know that funeral rituals repair the breach left by the dead. What we saw in New Orleans was a culture pushed beyond its capacity to mend the breach.

But only briefly. In a matter of weeks, the people of New Orleans went back to dealing with the dead. Again they improvised a kind of cultural rebuilding that seemed to draw on some of the ancient arts of being human. The professional handlers of the dead had been pushed past their limits, so some survivors dug graves for their dead relatives in city cemeteries that had lost all their low-paid workers. Relatives of the dead cut the weeds that grew between the graves when the city scrapped a plan to let prisoners work in cemeteries because no one wanted sickles, scythes, and weed whackers in the hands of felons. By the end of October 2005, the people of New Orleans were back in their cemeteries, ready for Halloween, and ready to tend graves. Reporters were happy to see them there and described the return of customs that colored life in New Orleans: children singing in a graveyard, mourners lighting votive candles and cleaning graves, or satirical Halloween revelers costumed in the blue tarps FEMA had used to cover corpses.[19]

In Robert Pogue Harrison's terms, such activities might be seen as signs of repossessing the city. "The surest way to take possession of a place and secure it as one's own is to bury one's dead in it," he points out. Not everyone behaves this way, he adds—nomadic peoples, for example. But in the modern West we bury our dead where we believe they belong. Relatives of some who died, exiled in Houston, worried that they could not properly bury their dead, as these family members might have been left in empty houses, misburied in debris, or covered by a tarp in the street. In New Orleans, possession of the city meant reburial of those to whom it belonged and hence a repossession of the city and a redeployment of the city's playful mix of voodoo and Catholicism. The news stories about Halloween and the cemeteries were meant to be reassuring.

The city's culture of the dead was coming back together, even if the city was not, and even if returning residents were still turning up rotting bodies in attics and trash piles. The horrible days of the promiscuous mixing of living and dead were coming to an end. The world began to resume its modern order.[20]

But can we put the memories of those promiscuous times to some good use, take orders from the ghosts we have seen? Joseph Roach describes a French naturalist named C. C. Robin who arrived in New Orleans in 1805, just after his country sold Louisiana to the United States. In one of the new government's first acts, authorities prohibited slaves from gathering in the city's public places. Crowds brewed rebellion. But authorities made an exception for funerals. Robin "noticed especially in the city that the funerals of white people are only attended by a few, those of colored people are attended by a great crowd, and mulattoes, quadroons, married to white people, do not disdain attending the funeral of a black." Death provided an occasion for a promiscuous assembly of the living. Did authorities assume that grief muted dreams of rebellion?[21]

If they did, they missed a point that the Bush administration knew all too well. Grief, uncontrolled and uncontained, can also be a catalyst to political action. Why else had our mourning become so scripted? Why else did the Bush administration make it so difficult for people to see even the coffins of the dead soldiers coming back from Iraq? Out of privacy and respect, they said. Perhaps the dead, briefly so very visible in New Orleans, can help us remember the hidden dead: both those Americans shipped back from Iraq or, more often, those lost Iraqis still in Iraq.

To act on our grief, we have to make politics out of scandal and shock and, strange as it seems, learn to remember the ghosts emanating from the unburied. The word that came up most often in reports of the discovery of the unburned bodies stacked in the Georgia woods was "scandal." The quick shorthand for the whole story became "the crematory scandal" or the "gruesome scandal." The court ordered the operator to apologize. States considered new regulatory legislation. People asked to watch bodies being inserted into crematories.[22] Shock and scandal over the unburned bodies hatched outrage that pushed for action. Can we keep the floating dead in New Orleans fresh as scandal, help the bodies retain their power to shock?

Another ghost might help. The association may seem odd, but those first images of bodies floating through New Orleans brought to mind an image of Ophelia painted by John Everett Millais in 1852. Drowned Ophelia floats in her watery grave. She invites sympathy. The dead who floated in the muck of the swollen canals of New Orleans ask for something more than sympathy. If we are to act for Katrina's dead, we might want to consider a different scene from *Hamlet*. It is Hamlet's father's ghost, or the apparition Hamlet imagines as his father's ghost that sets the play in motion. The ghost governs actions from beyond the grave. "Remember me," the ghost admonishes, and memory pushes

Hamlet to act. Katrina's ghosts call on us to remember, too. They also call on us to act, not with Hamlet's murderous vengeance, but as dutiful kinsmen to the city's survivors. Then our grief might have a point and a politics, and we might do something about the many mostly hidden things we glimpsed when the levees broke.

ACKNOWLEDGMENTS

I thank Rebecca Scales, Marc Matera, and Mel Stein for help on this essay.

NOTES

1. Norman Arey, "Guilty Plea in Huge Crematory Scandal," *Atlanta Journal-Constitution*, November 24, 2004, A1; Lori Andrews, "The Bones We Carried," *New York Times*, June 22, 2007, Op-Ed, A21.

2. Other chapters in this volume explore this story too. See Richard Mizelle Jr., "Second-Lining the Jazz City: Jazz Funerals, Katrina, and the Reemergence of New Orleans"; and Evie Shockley, "The Haunted Houses of New Orleans: Gothic Homelessness and African American Experience."

3. McCarthy quoted in Andrew Buncombe, "Hurricane Katrina: Memorial for Vera in the City Where the Dead Are Left Lying on the Streets," *Independent* (London), September 6, 2005, 2.

4. Matthew Brown, "Disturbed Rest," *Times-Picayune*, January 22, 2006, 1; the quote appears in a story by Gwen Filosa, "Body Hunt Continues in Lower 9th," *Times-Picayune*, "Metro," 1. On bodies coming out of coffins, see David Zucchino and Nicholas Riccardi, "Hurricane Dead Stuck in a Logistical Limbo," *Los Angeles Times*, October 10, 2005, A12.

5. Honoré quoted in Solomon Moore, David Zucchino, and Stephen Braun, "Katrina's Aftermath," *Los Angeles Times*, September 10, 2005, A1.

6. Walt Philbin, "Son Finds Body in Rubble," *Times-Picayune*, December 30, 2005, 1; Robert Travis Scott and Tara Young, "Bodies Still Being Found in Debris," *Times-Picayune*, October 23, 2005, 1; "Katrina Victim Found," *Toronto Sun*, May 29, 2006, 16; "Workers Find Body in Flooded Home," *Times-Picayune*, June 18, 2006, 1.

7. DMORT: Disaster Mortuary Operational Response Teams, http://www.dmort.org/DNPages/DMORTWhy.htm (accessed January 16, 2008); Shaila Dewan, "Storm and Crisis: The Dead," *New York Times*, September 29, 2005, A1.

8. Prayer quoted in Robert Travis Scott, "Recovery Chief Says Corpse Retrieval Lagged," *Times-Picayune*, September 15, 2005, News section, 1.

9. Nagin reference and Landrieu quote appear in Michelle Krupa, "Bodies Lie for Days Awaiting Retrieval," *Times-Picayune*, September 13, 2005, A1.

10. Blanco quoted in Michelle Krupa, "State Contracts to Remove Storm Dead," *Times-Picayune*, September 13, 2005.

11. Robert Pogue Harrison, *The Dominion of the Dead* (Chicago: University of Chicago Press, 2003), xi.

12. Robert Hertz, *Death and the Right Hand* (Glencoe, Ill.: Free Press, 1960), 27.

13. Available at http://www.georgewbush-whitehouse.archives.gov/news/releases/2005/09/20050910.html.

14. President Bush quoted in Christopher Rowland and Stephen Smith, "44 Found Dead in New Orleans Hospital," *Boston Globe*, September 13, 2005, A1.

15. Ibid.

16. Jackson quoted in Shaila Dewan, "In Attics and Rubble, More Bodies and Questions," *New York Times*, April 11, 2006, A1.

17. Ceci Connolly and Manuel Roig-Franzia, "Grim Map Details Toll in 9th Ward and Beyond: Katrina Proved Deadly in Every Section of New Orleans," *Washington Post*, October 23, 2005, A14; Coleman Warner and Robert Travis Scott, "Where They Died," *Times-Picayune*, October 23, 2005, 1.

18. Joseph Roach, *Cities of the Dead: Circum-Atlantic Performance* (New York: Columbia University Press, 1996), 15, 2.

19. Lynne Jensen, "With Cemetery Staff Scarce, New Orleans Families Fend for Themselves When It Comes to Burying Their Dead," *Times-Picayune*, July 23, 2006, 1; John Schwartz, "Archaeologist in New Orleans Finds a Way to Help the Living," *New York Times*, January 3, 2006, 1; Bruce Weber, "In New Orleans, Fewer Visitors Honor the Dead," *New York Times*, November 2, 2005, A26.

20. Harrison, *Dominion of the Dead*, 24; Lynne Jensen, "Solace in Silence," *Times-Picayune*, November 2, 2005, 1.

21. Roach, *Cities of the Dead*, 60.

22. Norman Arey, "Funeral Directors Review Crematory Procedures," *Atlanta Journal-Constitution*, July 5, 2002, 3D.

6

Second-Lining the Jazz City

Jazz Funerals, Katrina, and the Reemergence of New Orleans

RICHARD MIZELLE JR.

Jazz, along with blues, shrimp gumbo, po-boy sandwiches, world-famous steak-houses in the French Quarter, and tantalizing desserts like Mama's bread pudding and Café du Monde's beignets, came to symbolize the pulsating life of New Orleans. Accessible to ships from Africa, Europe, Asia, Latin America, and the Caribbean, the city's fusion of Spanish, West African, and European cultures shaped not only New Orleans's Creole identity but contributed to the evolution of jazz. The sound of jazz likely emerged out of the field hollers and spirituals developed by enslaved African peoples in the swamps, lowlands, fields, churches, and houses (away from the penetrating gaze of slaveholders) of the U.S. South.[1] Born of cultural exchange, early New Orleans jazz was a mixture of various musical genres, including blues, ragtime, and spirituals. Jazz consisted of a much wider range of musical instruments—including brass and reed instruments in particular—than the earlier piano ragtime bands. Improvisation and call and response became key elements of early jazz, creating space for individual and, in a broader sense, group expression.[2]

The history and culture of New Orleans is also closely linked with the jazz funeral, a unique and ritualized ceremony of mourning and celebration. The process of celebration and rejuvenation in a jazz funeral is called the "second line," and I use this term as a model for how we can apply the lessons of Katrina to bring change. The jazz funeral is both a metaphor for dealing with the losses caused by Katrina and a window into the culture of New Orleans. Jazz funerals offer a way of understanding the psychological and physical pain of bereavement in New Orleans and provide a model for the regeneration of the city and its people's spirits. I essentially make three points in this chapter, in relatively quick and short order. First, the history and resiliency of jazz funerals throughout the twentieth century is an important part of the people and culture of New Orleans. Second, many people have evoked the symbol of the jazz funeral to

69

describe the loss associated with Katrina, but loss is not only about death. The jazz funeral can provide an alternative lens for us to look at other, less measurable, concepts of deprivation and Katrina. Last is my theoretical use of second-lining and how we can apply this process in practical ways now. In these widened conceptions of loss, the theoretical concept of second-lining the jazz city becomes an important marker for affecting public policy.

The Jazz Funeral

Like jazz itself, the tradition of jazz funerals is a cultural hybrid uniquely embedded in the culture of New Orleans. As Jason Berry explains, the origins of the jazz funeral "lie in the colonial era, as French brass bands played in large processions honoring generals and politicians. At the same time, in a public park called Congo Square, African slaves gathered in large concentric circles, ring dances, honoring ancestral spirits. Gradually the two traditions came together—the line and the ring—creating a new form of burial ceremony."[3]

During a jazz funeral, a brass band traditionally awaits outside of the church or funeral home for the services to be completed, then begins to play processional or mournful music like "Nearer My God to Thee." Before older cemeteries in the city became full, the entire procession, including the band, would proceed to the gravesite. Now, because the newer sites are so far away, the family and close friends leave the band and people who have gathered to participate in or witness the jazz funeral. The band is usually led by a grand marshal, sometimes referred to as a "nelson," who is always a well-dressed gentleman. After a silence during which the band and crowd watch the deceased and family pass through the crowd, the body is then "cut loose" by the marshal, signaling the band to begin playing more upbeat music and the crowd to dance in a celebratory fashion. Mournful songs are replaced by tunes like "Didn't He Ramble."[4] As described by Joseph Roach, "cutting the body loose" to the spiritual world of heaven is less a forgetting of the deceased than a community replenishment toward the future and celebration of life.[5]

The dancers and marchers who follow the band as the entire scene moves through the streets of New Orleans are called the second line. These individuals are a unique component of this cultural performance, having at times various connections to the deceased and to a particular community. Although second-liners may know (even if not personally) well-known figures of New Orleans's musical scene celebrated with a jazz funeral, on other occasions second-liners may simply hear about or join in to celebrate the life of a local member of a community they did not know at all. Some second-liners bring their own brass instruments or drums and join in the band, while others elaborately decorate umbrellas that can be seen from blocks away. At the sight of a jazz funeral, people just walking on the street can join in the second line and participate in any way they see fit. The second line is a planned but spontaneous celebration of a community.

Customarily, it was well-respected local musicians or individuals affiliated with various fraternal and social clubs who were honored with a jazz funeral. Many of these social aid or pleasure clubs (as they were sometimes called) emerged in the decades after the Civil War. In addition to providing various social activities for their members, these clubs operated as insurance agencies for many African Americans in New Orleans, helping to defray medical and burial expenses for members, who paid weekly premiums. Social aid and benevolent clubs such as the Vidalia, Tulane, San Jacinto, and Jeunes Amis, for example, either had their own brass bands, drawn from among their members, or contracted a local band from New Orleans.[6]

The history of jazz funerals in New Orleans through the twentieth century is a macrocosm of cultural resiliency that reflects the microcosm of pain, hardships, and transformation that the people of New Orleans endured during and after Katrina. According to Ellis L. Marsalis Jr., who teaches jazz and piano at the University of New Orleans and is considered an authority on jazz funerals, brass bands through the 1920s played not only for funerals but for a wide range of other social functions as well, including weddings. Although Marsalis concedes that "the Great Depression severely hampered their activity . . . neither their music nor the playing of it for funerals passed from the scene."[7]

Yet Marsalis notes with some trepidation the transformation of jazz funerals in the past fifty years or so, as the older guard of jazz musicians in New Orleans have either retired or passed away. "Although the jazz funeral is very much a part of New Orleans' black culture, some of the younger brass band players are either unfamiliar with or indifferent to the traditional music. It is common to hear bands play popular songs of the day in place of the longtime standards handed down from the older musicians, and the stately march to the gravesite is becoming a thing of the past: often now the livelier music begins at the church door." The more modern bands were often independent of the social clubs, according to Marsalis, and instead of being exclusively reserved for musicians or club members, jazz funerals later could be secured by anyone willing to pay, reflecting a certain commoditization of jazz funeral culture.[8] So, although sightseeing is not the basis of this chapter, it is important to bring up briefly the tensions between tourism and jazz culture in New Orleans. Jazz is a point of contact between the city's natives and tourists. The dichotomy between jazz musicians' cultural contributions and the extraction of this culture and art for tourist revenue thus presents a complication in the story of the city's relationship to jazz. The lived experiences of musicians may tell part of the tale. For the average musician, finding a working gig in New Orleans has been a notoriously difficult task, alternating between low-paying jobs and unpaid jobs. Yet, visitors are bombarded with the images of jazz funerals in souvenir shops throughout the French Quarter. One sign reads, "Jazz Funerals: Where People Are Dying to Come In—New Orleans." The musicians of New Orleans, like other residents, are struggling to rebuild their lives and disconnected families, as well as to find places to play and work in a market where many venues have still not returned.

Evaluating Loss and Displacement

Jazz funerals in New Orleans are suggestive of the many perspectives of loss and the resiliency of a city and a culture. That this resiliency is linked to jazz is an idea that the city's own coroner has recognized for decades. Called by many "the trumpet-playing coroner of New Orleans," Frank "Jazz" Minyard, who has served for more than thirty years, demonstrates how much jazz is embedded in every aspect of New Orleans society and culture. Before Katrina, visitors to the official Web site of the coroner's office were greeted with sounds of jazz.[9] After Katrina, Minyard continued to place jazz alongside loss when he appeared with Melissa Block on National Public Radio's *All Things Considered* program on October 17, 2005. The coroner, who himself plays in a band, told Block, "a couple of weeks ago, I hadn't practiced or played because of the hurricane, and I took out my trumpet in the quiet place of my trailer and I played 'Do You Know What It Means to Miss New Orleans?' and I started crying. The devastation, not only of the place, but of the people, and our lives, none of us will ever be the same, ever." He then sang the first verse of Louis Armstrong's classic homage to the city, "Do you know what it means to miss New Orleans, and miss it each night and day?"[10]

Ann Fabian discusses the complex meanings of Katrina's dead in her chapter. It is very true that, in the words of Katherine Verdery, dead bodies have "political lives." The living often attach their own meanings to the dead, who are no longer able to voice their own feelings of anger, frustration, dismay, success, or failure. Politicized death can be a powerful phenomenon and is not always linear. Death can lead to a reinterpretation of an individual's life in interesting ways.[11] The deaths of Katrina victims are stories of neglect and displacement in life as well as death. It is how we remember these dead that may provide the most powerful critique of Katrina, historically and in the form of public policy. But, the tale of Katrina and loss is about more than the dead. It is also about the survivors and their losses. Many have argued that the Katrina's dead were forgotten by society before and after the storm, victims of structural inequality and poverty. In similar ways, survivors and their experiences can easily be forgotten as well.

Katrina is a symbol of loss, not only of life and property, but of things immeasurable to many of us. Scholars and the public in general often attempt to assign numbers to what is in many ways resistant to reduction. The destruction of homes, which are such an important component of economic capital in this country, surely was devastating, not just in the short run but in the long run as well. Historically, many people in this country have to build wealth and equity from "scratch" or nothing. For many in New Orleans, the loss of these homes will affect future generations, as this property would have been passed down to children and grandchildren, making the loss of homes particularly disheartening for economically poorer people who have scraped for a generation to buy and maintain a home. Yet we often make the mistake of overlooking what was inside the home. Reductionist concepts that provide monetary figures for property damage losses do not take into account the loss of, for example, the family Bible that recorded your baptism as a child, the pocket watch your father gave you, or the countless pictures of relatives lining the wall or in photo albums that are part of your existence.[12] The loss of these artifacts and personal belongings is more than just an unfortunate circumstance of disaster; for many this is the disaster. Physically and psychologically this loss will affect survivors for the remainder of their lives. And it can be equally difficult to measure loss of life, given that the pain and suffering experienced through Katrina may take a toll on survivors well into the next decade and longer.

But, perhaps a better way to look at it is through the term "displacement." I ask my students sometimes, "What is the difference between displacement and migration?" In the aftermaths of both the Great Mississippi Flood of 1927 and Katrina, many survivors were displaced from their land and homes and migrated to cities in the urban South and the North. Displacement can have another meaning, though, equally linked to the idea of loss. The loss of neighborhood familiarity, support networks, longtime health-care providers, or something as seemingly banal as the neighborhood market where you bought fresh fish every Friday morning all constitute displacement. This kind of displacement operates as sort of an internal revolution or unsettling that sufferers do not often talk about. The elderly, particularly those eighty-five and older, can suffer tremendously from a breakdown of social networks and familiarity. Outliving family and friends and losing the personal possessions that provided comfort, as well as the support structure of the community, can take a enormous toll on this population in disasters such as Katrina. This emotional and psychological distress, I would argue, can lead to or exacerbate physical ailments.[13]

Second-Lining the Jazz City

In the midst of all of this pain and loss, where can the city and America look for rejuvenation? In *Cities of the Dead*, Joseph Roach describes non-Western ceremonies of death in the circum-Atlantic world as an empowerment of "the living through the performance of memory."[14] The performances, he argues, are not only for the deceased but also for the loss and renewal of the community's cohesiveness and spirit. These celebrations serve to mourn death and cata-strophic events in the community. But in "cutting loose" those catastrophic events mourners also look toward the future. These spirit-world ceremonies in some non-Western contexts are part of a continuum in the relationship of the living with ancestors. An early product of New Orleans's own musical ancestors, the jazz funeral forms such a ceremony that itself cuts loose and looks forward.[15]

After Katrina, some have said that New Orleans is dead, that it will never return to the way it was. My concern is less whether it will return (for I think it will) than how it will return, and who will be involved in the process and in what ways. The tradition of jazz funerals has become a popular symbol of loss and the celebration of culture in New Orleans in the years following Katrina, capturing the attention of a number of artists and filmmakers. Spike Lee's documentary, *When the Levees Broke: A Requiem in Four Acts*, opens with Armstrong's plaintive song. New Orleans's Dirty Dozen Brass Band's 2006 album, *What's Going On?*, frames Katrina as one event in a series of bewildering disasters the world has faced in recent years and uses the strong influence of the jazz funeral that marked its earlier album, *Funeral for a Friend*, in 2004. This album was dedicated to Anthony "Tuba Fats" Lacen, one of the founders of the Dirty Dozen Brass Band and a jazz icon on the musical landscape of New Orleans, who died of heart failure in 2004.

The particular quality of the jazz funeral that intrigues me, however, is found in Roach's suggestion that "the jazz funeral's genius for participation resides in the very expandability of the procession: marchers with very different connections to the deceased (or perhaps no connections at all) join together on the occasion to make connections with one another."[16] The theory of second-lining, then, provides a useful model for the rebuilding of New Orleans. We will need a "second line," in the traditional jazz funeral sense of people coming together from different backgrounds and agendas to influence present and future policy. Though we may not know New Orleans as our own home, like those in the second line who do not know the deceased, the appreciation that New Orleans is somebody's home can push a wide variety of people to remem-ber Katrina and New Orleans and work together.

As an example, in the years since Katrina, America has learned many les-sons from this disaster. Through Katrina, scholars have taken the opportunity to develop interdisciplinary alliances and conversations evident in edited col-lections like the present one. Within this volume are contributions from schol-ars representing history, political science, human ecology, public policy, and English literature. We are the theoretical second-liners coming together from different backgrounds, and our interactions and conversations can move our understanding of Katrina forward, and most important, seek significant policy change. The interdisciplinary nature of emerging scholarship can potentially influence public policy decisions.

Innovative courses are emerging on university campuses throughout the country on Katrina and the history of environmental disasters. Valuable teaching tools, like *Teaching the Levees: A Curriculum for Democratic Dialogues and Civic Engagement* (2007) through Columbia University's Teachers College, are now emerging. Along with a two-DVD set of Spike Lee's *When the Levees Broke*, the Teachers College, with support from the Rockefeller Foundation and HBO Documentary Films, produced an instructional guide for discussing Katrina on the high school and university levels, reflecting in its curriculum the need for interdisciplinary ideas.

Yet, the theoretical second-lining of academics from various disciplines hinges on a future trajectory and an uneasy activism in the realm of politics. Scholars are often uncomfortable in thinking of why and how their work can influence policy. Historian of medicine Charles Rosenberg eloquently describes this tension and the commonly held assumption "that historians should look backward, while the essence of policy is to look forward—as though the past is not in the present and the present in the future."[17] The power of theoretically second-lining the jazz city is that it has brought people together, exchanging ideas and interacting in ways they may have ordinarily never done. This is true in a traditional jazz funeral sense of people with seemingly little or no connection at all setting aside affiliations and restraints and coming together for the community. Key issues of transportation and immobility rooted in poverty, special needs of medically dependent populations, planning and infrastructure of houses and city services, evacuation management, resources for aging populations, just to name a few, can be greatly influenced by the scholarship of historians, urban planners, sociologists, and the medical humanities. Second-lining is about preparing intelligently for the future.

Katrina's story is powerful in that it presents an opportunity for change. Emergencies often bring about reevaluation of policies. In the aftermath of the rash of school shootings in recent years, secondary school systems and universities have reevaluated their emergency plans. After the Virginia Tech shooting in 2007, campuses nationwide developed new emergency protocols and warning systems. As one example of the Katrina effect, hospitals and nursing homes throughout the country have revisited the rules and guidelines to be followed in case of environmental disasters or other emergencies. A few of the questions addressed are when to evacuate patients, who makes the decision to evacuate, and how we can better keep track of medical records during an evacuation as people are scattered to other cities and states.

I hope these conversations will continue to occur and that perspectives and viewpoints from many disciplines will be incorporated into discussions of how present inequalities can be addressed and a future Katrina-like disaster averted. If the history of environmental disasters in America tells us anything, it is that memories are short.[18] People move on with life and more pressing issues. This is particularly true for those whom a disaster does not impact personally. The memories of Katrina's dead that Ann Fabian discusses should always be with us, as should the loss and struggles of survivors—some displaced even in New Orleans while others resettled in other parts of the country.

For the moment, though, why don't we let Armstrong's song play out as a remembrance of the people absented through death and migration from a city's landscape, as well as the pain and suffering of Katrina's survivors?

Do you know what it means to miss New Orleans
And miss it each night and day?
I know I'm not wrong . . . this feeling's getting stronger
The longer I stay away.
Miss them moss-covered vines . . . the tall sugar pines
Where mockingbirds used to sing
And I'd like to see that lazy Mississippi . . . . hurrying into spring.
The moonlight on the bayou. . . . a creole tune. . . . that fills the air
I dream. . . . about magnolias in bloom. . . . and I'm wishin' I was there.
Do you know what it means to miss New Orleans
When that's where you left your heart?
And there's one thing more . . . I miss the one I care for
More. . . . more than I miss. . . . New Orleans.[19]

Perhaps Gralen B. Banks tied it together best as he connected the culture of New Orleans with the loss of Katrina, showing why we should work so hard for the people of New Orleans to incorporate the history and lessons of Katrina into present and future decision making. He describes, with an unyielding pride of a soul born and raised in New Orleans, what it means when "your first breath when the doctor slapped you is tinted with magnolia blossoms and you drink Mississippi River tap water. Folks who had to evacuate know you might go somewhere and you might have a good time, but it's nothing like home. And when you can call New Orleans, Louisiana, home, baby, you know what it means to miss New Orleans, trust me."[20]

NOTES

1. Lawrence W. Levine, *Black Culture and Black Consciousness: Afro-American Folk Thought from Slavery to Freedom* (New York: Oxford University Press, 1977), 221–222.

2. Lewis Erenberg, *Swingin' the Dream: Big Band Jazz and the Rebirth of American Culture* (Chicago: University of Chicago Press, 1998), 3–35.

3. "Jazz Funerals," Religion and Ethics News Weekly, PBS online, http://www.pbs.org/wnet/religionandethics/week722/feature.html.

4. Gerald Early, "'And I Will Sing of Joy and Pain for You': Louis Armstrong and the Great Jazz Traditions; A Review-Essay," *Callaloo* 21 (1984): 90–100; Gary Donaldson, "A Window on Slave Culture: Dances at Congo Square in New Orleans, 1800–1862," *Journal of Negro History* 69, no. 2 (1984): 63–72.

5. Joseph Roach, *Cities of the Dead: Circum-Atlantic Performance* (New York: Columbia University Press, 1996), 277–281.

6. Leo Touchet and Vernel Bagneris, *Rejoice When You Die: The New Orleans Jazz Funerals* (Baton Rouge: Louisiana State University Press, 1998). This is a photography book; see the introduction by Ellis L. Marsalis Jr.

7. Marsalis introduction in Touchet and Bagneris, *Rejoice When You Die.*

8. Ibid.

9. Steven Gray and Evan Perez, *Wall Street Journal*, September 9, 2005.

10. National Public Radio News, *All Things Considered*, October 17, 2005. The interview was conducted by Melissa Block. "Do You Know What It Means to Miss New Orleans?" was written by Eddie DeLange and Louis Alter. The song was part of the original soundtrack of the 1947 movie *New Orleans*, where it was performed by Louis Armstrong and Billie Holiday.

11. See Katherine Verdery, *The Political Lives of Dead Bodies: Reburial and Postsocialist Change* (New York: Columbia University Press, 1999).

12. For an interesting discussion of memory and meaning as they relate to photographs and family artifacts in African American life and culture, see Cheryl A. Wall, *Worrying the Line: Black Women Writers, Lineage, and Literary Tradition* (Chapel Hill: University of North Carolina Press, 2005).

13. A recent work that discusses the particular vulnerability of the elderly in environmental disasters is Eric Klinenberg's *Heat Wave: A Social Autopsy of Disaster in Chicago* (Chicago: University of Chicago Press, 2002).

14. Roach, *Cities of the Dead*, 1–4.

15. Ibid.

16. Ibid., 279.

17. Charles E. Rosenberg, *Our Present Complaint: American Medicine, Then and Now* (Baltimore: Johns Hopkins University Press, 2007), 202–203.

18. For an excellent synthetic history of environmental disasters, see Ted Steinberg's *Acts of God: The Unnatural History of Natural Disaster in America* (New York: Oxford University Press, 2000).

19. Lyrics from "Do You Know What It Means to Miss New Orleans?" written by Eddie De Lange and Louis Alter © 1946 (renewed 1974, 2002) De Lange Music Co. (ASCAP)/ administered by Bug Music and Louis Alter Music Publications, New York. All rights outside the United States controlled by Edwin H. Morris & Company, a division of MPL Music Publishing, Inc. All rights reserved. Used by permission.

20. Gralen B. Banks is director of security at the Hyatt Regency in New Orleans and was interviewed in Spike Lee's *When the Levees Broke* (40 Acres and a Mule Filmworks Production, 2006).

7

Racism, Trauma, and Resilience

The Psychological Impact of Katrina

NANCY BOYD-FRANKLIN

Since Katrina, I have worked with hurricane survivors and have trained mental health providers treating the victims of this catastrophic event. I have traveled to New Orleans and other cities in Louisiana and Mississippi and have been profoundly affected by the destruction that I witnessed as well as the psychological trauma experienced by so many African Americans. Victims confronted multiple levels of trauma: the hurricane itself; the displacement of thousands when the levees broke; the desperation of waiting for help that was long overdue—whether on rooftops or in unendurable conditions in the Superdome or the Convention Center, with no food or water for days. Many witnessed death and destruction, including bloated dead bodies floating in the floodwaters. As I have traveled throughout this country and have spoken to African American survivors of Katrina, they express a profound sense of sadness and loss that Linda Burton and colleagues have described as a deep and painful yearning and psychological longing for their home.[1] Even those who have remained in or returned to their city have been overwhelmed by the surreal experience of viewing the destruction and devastation that is still everywhere in the Lower Ninth Ward and other historically black communities.

This chapter examines the multiple dimensions of the psychological trauma produced by Hurricane Katrina—both for the victims of the storm and for a broader African American community. To understand the ways in which trauma was produced, we must understand two things. First is how the trauma fed on historically created vulnerabilities. As others have demonstrated in this volume, blacks faced greater likelihood of experiencing various hardships associated with the disaster and the aftermath owing to their preexisting economic and social vulnerabilities. Second, a fairly consistent message emerged from events and media coverage of the storm: that black Americans were not full citizens of America. Enshrined in law for much of American history and recapitulated during Katrina, this message became a prominent feature of the hurricane. Throughout American history, blacks have shown resilience in adapting to this reality by creating alternative support systems (homes, churches, and community institutions). Hurricane Katrina swept many of these supports away and exposed the fragility of worth and belonging that has long defined the African American experience. This chapter examines the psychological impact, this history, and the ongoing story of African American resilience.

In a world that is often a very dangerous place for black people, "home" becomes a refuge, or as bell hooks (and Evie Shockley, in this volume) has described it, as a safe place where African Americans could "be affirmed in our minds and hearts despite poverty, hardship, and deprivation, where we could restore to ourselves the dignity denied us on the outside in the public world."[2] In this context, home is not just a house; it is a communal web of familiarity, safety, and love that protected many victims of Katrina for many generations. It was this profound sense of "home" or "homeplace" that many African Americans have lost in the aftermath of the storm.[3] Media commentators were largely unaware of the cultural significance of home or homeplace to many African American residents. This home may have been passed down through generations and the only possession of value that they had in the world. For many, this was not just the loss of their family home, but their communities, their church homes, and the close, communal network of people who made up their blood and nonblood "families."[4]

Trauma faced by so many was a complex, overdetermined experience that included (1) the hurricane-related trauma of the physical dislocation and loss of life and property and (2) the effects of racism and classism in the post-Katrina response that was visible to far more observers than merely the victims. As an African American woman and a psychologist, even as I watched in horror in August 2005 as television coverage of the aftermath of Hurricane Katrina revealed thousands of black people being treated with the most extreme forms of disrespect and racism, I saw these events as part of a larger story of race and trauma. The message of the coverage was also striking for what it revealed about belonging, blame, and deservingness: who belongs to America, who is to blame for racial inequality, and who deserves to be rescued. Given this reality, the ensuing and continuing absence of appropriate governmental response and the lack of ongoing outcry from the mental health professions have been even more appalling.

With Katrina, the physical threats to African American bodies became long-lasting psychological burdens. But Katrina also exposed another feature of the black experience: survival and resilience. The second part of this chapter will discuss the resilience of survivors and the cultural strengths that have sustained them. The African American survivors of Katrina whom I have met have often asked only one thing of me— "Please write about our experiences so that America does not forget us." Here, I am honoring that promise.

Hurricane Katrina: Double Psychological Trauma and Media Coverage

Victims of Hurricane Katrina experienced a double psychological trauma: the first was the topic of extensive coverage; the second has not been examined in great detail. The first trauma arose directly from the hurricane and included the death, loss, and separation from family and extended family members; the loss of their homes and all of their possessions; and the loss of their sense of beloved community, with its own unique culture. The second psychological trauma, which concerns me in this chapter, stemmed from the sense (felt by African Americans nationwide) that neglect was rooted in racism and classism. Subsequent analyses (including several chapters in this volume) have documented that racism and classism left many poor African Americans extraordinarily vulnerable in New Orleans and other areas affected by Katrina.[5] That the unimaginable neglect was visible as a nationwide event—epitomized by images of thousands of African Americans fleeing deplorable conditions with no food or water for five days at the Superdome and the Convention Center—clearly led to double psychological trauma, race-related stress, and physical and emotional hardship for the survivors, and vicariously experienced trauma for African Americans elsewhere.[6] Of course, many Americans (regardless of race) were shocked by the horrifying conditions television cameras revealed, but extensive media coverage spun the images as the disclosure of an unspoken truth that reflected the reality of race and poverty in America—the 67 percent of New Orleans residents who were black and poor.[7]

The media coverage often generated and framed racialized images that accentuated the trauma for African Americans. One particularly telling example was the contrasting captions on two photographs capturing a similar event in the struggle to survive: a lone black man pulling a plastic bag through the water and a white couple pushing a shopping cart full of groceries. The caption under the picture of the black man read: "A young [black] man walks through chest-deep flood water after looting a grocery store in New Orleans" while the caption under the picture of the white couple read, "Two [white] residents wade through chest-deep water after finding bread and soda from a local grocery store."[8] The African American victims of the storm were often characterized by the media in these pejorative ways.[9] Stereotypes of African Americans as looters were repeated throughout the coverage.

The language used to describe African Americans who were forced to relocate was not only problematic but also had traumatic effects. Initially, news organizations described individuals who were forced to relocate and find shelter as "refugees."[10] In his extensive analysis of the media coverage in the first week after the hurricane hit, linguist Geoffrey Nunberg found that in articles where the words "poor" and "black" appeared, the term "refugee" was more likely to be used than "evacuee."[11] Samuel Sommers and colleagues argue that "these data support the conclusion that race played some role in the use of 'refugee' in the coverage of Katrina."[12] African American leaders throughout the country objected to this term and contended that it was racially biased because it "depicted the Black population in outgroup terms and implied that the victims were less than full citizens."[13] After the understandable uproar about this vocabulary, the words "evacuees," "survivors," or "victims" were substituted for "refugees."

Adding further to our understanding of psychological trauma, the Sommers article also identified an emphasis on violent crime in media discussions of African American survivors as a group.[14] Although much of the reporting on snipers, gunfire, homicides, gangs of youth roaming the city, rapes, and so forth was later proven false, the images endured. Interestingly, coverage of predominantly white, middle-class areas did not include these stereotypic references to violence—it was only mentioned in the coverage of areas such as the Superdome and the Convention Center, which housed large numbers of African Americans. Tragically, this misreporting kept some individuals from following through on rescue efforts.[15] The embedded racism found in media reporting on Katrina is nothing new. Research by Robert Entman and Andrew Rojecki has documented that in many cases historically, "media coverage of Blacks disproportionately emphasizes violent crime."[16]

The infamous events in Gretna (a white community near New Orleans, which repelled evacuees) demonstrate the concrete origins and effects of such media images. Kristin Henkel, John Dovidio, and Samuel Gaertner describe this disturbing incident:

> [O]n September 1, 2005, 3 days after Hurricane Katrina struck, thousands of evacuees who were fleeing the wretched conditions of the city and the Convention Center marched toward a bridge that would take them to safety [in the predominately white community of Gretna]. They were met at the bridge by Gretna Police who brandished rifles. The evacuees recount hearing gunshots [fired over their heads] . . . as the police prevented them from crossing the bridge and turned them back toward the city. Two visitors trying to escape New Orleans wrote about their experiences: "We questioned why we couldn't cross the bridge. . . . They responded that the West Bank was not going to become New Orleans and there would be no Superdome in their city." . . . The police chief explained that "his town feared for its safety from a tide of evacuees."[17]

At the same time, the media documented other incidents of racism and racial stereotyping that further victimized African American survivors and "fueled racial suspicions and exacerbated racial mistrust."[18] And, as Aaron Sharockman observed about the Gretna event, "because most of the evacuees were Black and most of Gretna is White, the episode has stirred charges of racism."[19] But simply to call it racism is to ignore a more fundamental question of what type of racism this is, and how racism can exist outside of the conscious awareness of whites.

Different Types of Racism and Trauma

Black and white Americans interpreted images from Katrina—thousands of people left with no food or water for days on end, crying out for help—very differently.[20] A CNN/USA Today Poll conducted approximately two weeks after Katrina, on September 13, 2005, asked respondents whether race was a factor in the slow response to Katrina victims. Sixty percent of blacks viewed race as a factor, while only 12 percent of whites did. Some white Americans depict inequities as arising from "class not race."[21] A vast majority of whites polled even denied that class was a factor in the slow response to Katrina. When participants were asked if the poverty of the victims was a factor in the slow response, 63 percent of blacks saw this as a factor, while only 21 percent of whites gave a similar response. These results should not be surprising; polls have consistently documented a similar pattern.

Within the past ten years there has been a growing body of research studies documenting the psychological trauma of perceived racism and demonstrating that racism need not be proven "objectively" in order to produce psychological stress and emotional trauma.[22] This observation helps to explain the divergence in the polling results about racial perceptions and calls attention to a prominent debate in the psychological literature concerning African Americans' perceptions of racism.[23] Such perceptions, particularly in terms of their psychological impact, were discounted in discussions of racism. This has been especially true in the past thirty years, when blatant racism and segregation were replaced with more subtle forms that could be easily denied.[24] Clearly, the results of the CNN poll indicate that a majority of African American respondents perceived racism and classism in the aftermath of Katrina, and this added to the psychological trauma for many of the survivors.[25]

Katrina is an example of not one but many different kinds of racism. As Peggy McIntosh, a noted white feminist, has shown, many white Americans view racism as individual acts of meanness.[26] But there is another even more insidious form of racism that exists on an institutional level. Institutional racism is far more pervasive, and it is so embedded in the fabric of America that it is often "invisible" to those who are not directly affected by it.[27] It is reflected in the historical disparities in the treatment of blacks and whites in New Orleans and in many other parts of America. These differences were reflected in the chronic, long-term poverty of many of the African Americans living in New Orleans.

Pre-Katrina, 67 percent of New Orleans was black and poor.[28] Examples of the chronic, contextual stress of racism[29] associated with Katrina include the multi-generational nature of the extreme poverty experienced by many black people living in New Orleans's Lower Ninth Ward, which were among the most devastated areas.[30]

As many scholars have established, both individual and institutional forms of racism often operate outside of the conscious awareness of whites and may not involve direct intention to harm blacks. My intention here is to draw attention to the interactions between these forms of racism, as well as their psychological effects. Michael Eric Dyson, in his compelling book on Katrina, argues that "although one may not have racial intent, one's actions may nonetheless have racial consequences."[31] Henkel, Dovidio, and Gaertner make a similar case and define institutional racism as "the intentional or unintentional manipulation or toleration of institutional policies . . . that unfairly restrict the opportunities of particular groups of people."[32] Implicit in this point is the notion that institutional racism involves psychological processes. They further contend that "historical discrimination against Blacks produces a legal disparity that may be perpetuated even by well-intentioned people who endorse and exercise current policies that have disparate consequences for Whites and Blacks."[33] Given these realities, Henkel and coauthors indicate that "when a racial group and its members have been historically disadvantaged, the consequences are broad and severe, reproducing themselves across time."[34] For example, authorities were aware that the Ninth Ward, the area in which many poor African Americans lived, was highly susceptible to flooding in the event of a major hurricane, but no preventive steps were taken to avoid this disaster.[35] Thus, these multiple types of racism and classism (evident in policies that segregated and contributed to generations of poverty in the lives of many of the African American residents of the New Orleans) were in place long before Hurricane Katrina struck, and they played a part in the disregard for the personal welfare of the disproportionate number of African Americans who experienced the catastrophic impact of the storm and the post-Katrina events.

Psychological research has continually deepened our understanding of racism, embedded in large- and small-scale events. Shelly Harrell identifies six types of race-related psychological stressors, all of which can be recognized in the experiences of the African Americans who were impacted by Hurricane Katrina: (1) *Racism-related life events* were experienced by thousands of black people during and after Hurricane Katrina, and this framework of analysis might help us to understand the Gretna story. (2) *Vicarious racism experiences* were felt by many African Americans throughout the country who watched in horror as "their people" were allowed to fester in deplorable conditions, and this phenomenon could help us to understand the polling differences. (3) *Microaggressions* is a term that refers to the daily experiences of slights, exclusion, abandonment, and disrespect evident in the experience of many African American Katrina survivors, quite a few of whom live now outside their home communities, forced to rely on strangers. Psychological studies have barely begun to look closely at these microaggressions. (4) *Chronic contextual stress* is the term by which Harrell describes the societal structural inequities that existed for generations in the extreme poverty of many African Americans in New Orleans and other parts of the Gulf region. It was vividly evident in the thousands of predominantly black faces at the Convention Center and at the Superdome in New Orleans, and it is also evident in the challenge of rebuilding lives post-Katrina. (5) *Collective trauma*—whenever something as disturbing as Hurricane Katrina and the racism of the response occurs, it is experienced collectively by black people because of the collective nature of African American culture. (6) *Transgenerational transmission of stress and trauma* associated with the legacy of racism in this country, which includes slavery, oppression, Jim Crow laws, segregation, discrimination, poverty, and the brutality of the treatment of black demonstrators during the civil rights movement.[36] Clearly, Katrina provided Americans with an opportunity to understand this complex phenomenon called racism. Fundamentally, the question of racism evokes questions of trust. It has been well documented that African Americans have learned to distrust many aspects of their experience in America and have developed a mechanism, which I have labeled "healthy cultural suspicion," that has helped them to survive.[37] The images of Hurricane Katrina have been deeply ingrained on the psyche of many African Americans, and there is no question that the experiences of racism during the storm have reinforced this healthy suspicion.[38]

To what extent did Katrina-related racism contribute to post-traumatic stress disorder (PTSD) in black Americans?[39] The field of psychology has resisted acknowledging racism as a contributing factor to PTSD in African Americans and other persons of color, despite research, discussed above, documenting that racism can be a form of psychological trauma for this population independent of the material effects of racism.[40]

This analysis of psychological trauma and race adds considerably to our understanding of vulnerability in America—complementing other chapters in this volume on transportation, health care, and environmental vulnerabilities. This chapter suggests that the effects of Katrina were not isolated to the displaced Gulf Coast population of African Americans. Katrina helps us to identify a far-reaching psychological vulnerability with concrete implications for African Americans' place in American society. Indeed, Niki Dickerson's chapter in the following section can be read as extending this analysis—with its discussion of the resistance that evacuees found as they attempted to establish new homes in new neighborhoods.

Unquestionably, however, stress was a crucial part of the Katrina experience. Research by James Elliott and Jeremy Pais on 1,200 Katrina survivors showed that blacks generally reported higher levels of stress than whites.[41] In addition to the agonizing traumas of seeing their loved ones die, of prolonged separation without word of their safety, and of stressful, life-threatening conditions, African American survivors of Katrina were subjected to other distresses that were related to the racism and racial indignities that they endured. News reports from that period are full of poignant pleas from African American survivors, who felt that their country had abandoned them because of their race.[42] This was the lesson of Katrina for many African Americans nationwide.

The Trauma and Disparities Continue

The disparities I have discussed thus far are further complicated by the significance of the loss of home and community for many blacks, who because of the long legacy of racism and segregation have viewed their homes as sanctuaries in an oppressive environment. That illusive sense of safety has now disappeared for many African American survivors. Ronald Kessler of Harvard Medical School has completed one of the most comprehensive surveys of the mental health of Hurricane Katrina survivors from Louisiana, Mississippi, and Alabama.[43] The study found that the proportion of people with a serious mental illness doubled in the months after Katrina compared with a survey conducted several years before. The study found that despite this dramatic increase in mental illness, suicidal thoughts did not increase. Kessler expressed concerns that this decrease in reports of suicidal ideation might be associated with unrealistically high hopes for the recovery efforts. He expressed concern that these reports of suicidal feelings might increase if the anticipated help was not provided.[44] This is clearly a concern as time passes, as many of the survivors continue to experience bureaucratic red tape and broken promises.

A Kaiser Family Foundation study, based on house-to-house interviews of 1,504 survivors of Hurricane Katrina who remained in or returned to New Orleans, reported that eight in ten individuals have seen a deterioration in their quality of life in areas such as economic well-being, access to health care, physical and mental health issues, lack of employment or low wages, or having a child in need of medical or mental health care that is not available.[45] These researchers note that their findings may underestimate the devastation of the hurricane because only about half of the pre-Katrina population of 484,674 currently lives in New Orleans.

Kaiser Family Foundation president and CEO Drew Altman stated that the study found a "huge and significant racial divide in the city" and that African

Americans were "hit much harder." He also indicated that blacks in Orleans Parish were disproportionately affected after Katrina:

> Twice as many African Americans as whites in Orleans [Parish] (59 per-cent vs. 29 percent) reported that their lives are still "very" or "some-what" disrupted. African Americans within Orleans were significantly more likely than Orleans whites (58 percent vs. 34 percent) to live in areas that experienced heavy flooding. In addition, seven in ten African Americans in Orleans Parish (72 percent) reported a problem accessing health care, more than twice the rate reported by whites in the parish (32 percent). African Americans in the city also reported more often than their white neighbors that their financial situation had gotten worse, that they had no job or earned too little, or that they had a child facing a health-care related problem. There were also striking differences in the ways that blacks and whites in Orleans Parish view the recovery efforts. More than half (55 percent) of blacks in the parish said that they face worse treatment and opportunities than whites as a part of the rebuild-ing process; among white Orleans residents, only 19 percent said blacks are being treated worse.[46]

Janet Ruscher has indicated that "many of the same people stranded by Katrina's floodwaters remain stranded by bureaucratic inertia, institutional-ized inequity, and inadequate mental health services."[47] Survivors continue to live in appalling conditions, including "overcrowding, delay in delivery [of government-provided trailers], failure to attach utilities, denial of assistance, dangerous surroundings, and constant threats of discontinuance of housing."[48] This was particularly evident in the case of the sixty thousand families in Louisiana who, as of 2006, still resided in 240-square-foot trailers provided by Federal Emergency Management Agency (FEMA), usually with a minimum of three other family members. Even eighteen months after Katrina, over half of the homes in New Orleans's African American communities still did not have electricity and over half of the population had still not returned.[49]

These realities are further complicated for New Orleans's black and poor former residents, who are now displaced in cities and other communities across the country. Prior to Katrina, many were renters, often living in low-income housing developments. There is an "urgent need for 30,000 affordable rental apartments in New Orleans alone—another 15,000 around the rest of the state."[50] The loss of affordable housing has been acutely felt in poor black areas of the city, where more than "80 percent of the 5,100 New Orleans occupied public housing apartments remained closed by order of the U.S. Department of Housing and Urban Development (HUD)."[51] In many white areas of the city, it is clear that poor black residents are not welcome.[52] Similarly, many of the urban renewal plans call for the replacement of low-income housing developments with mixed-income housing that will increase the likelihood that former poor black residents will not be able to return.[53]

In addition, many black homeowners in the Ninth Ward did not have sufficient insurance coverage to allow them to rebuild their homes.[54] All of these realities contribute to the loss of a significant number of African American residents of New Orleans. These losses have impacted Katrina survivors of many different racial and ethnic groups, but they have clearly disproportionately affected poor African Americans.

Resilience

What has allowed black Americans to weather the storm and the aftermath as they have? How have African Americans coped with these multiple levels of racism and psychological trauma associated with displacement, microaggressions, and media-generated vicarious racism? Throughout history, generations of African Americans have maintained their human dignity and have demonstrated multiple levels of resilience, determination, and survival skills in the face of many atrocities and assaults on their humanity, such as slavery, the Middle Passage, Jim Crow laws, segregation, lynching, overt and covert racism, discrimination, stereotyping, and now, Hurricane Katrina. Religious faith and spirituality has been a major source of resilience and survival skills for African Americans historically and a way to heal from the losses and indignities they have suffered from in this country, such as brutal treatment, oppression, racism, and disaster situations. Some African Americans express psychological distress in spiritual terms. In psychotherapy, African Americans will often use spiritual metaphors to express survival and psychological resilience. I have enumerated many examples of spiritual metaphors that can be very helpful to clinicians.[55] For example, in desperate times, such as during Hurricane Katrina and when facing death, many African Americans will recite Psalm 23 from the Bible: "Though I walk through the valley of the shadow of death, I shall fear no evil, for Thou art with me."

For African Americans, resilience has been rooted in spirituality and religious beliefs. These beliefs often serve a psychological function and promote positive mental health.[56] This reliance on spirituality and faith has a long history for black people. I have demonstrated the ways in which it is deeply ingrained in the culture and provides support and comfort, particularly in times of disruption, loss, and grief, such as Katrina. A research study conducted by Elliott and Pais showed important differences in black and white Katrina survivors in terms of how they viewed and prioritized their spirituality and religious faith. Whites were much more likely to report relying on families or friends during and in the aftermath of Katrina, whereas reliance on religious faith was reported more often by blacks. Interestingly, although many blacks reported staying in the homes of family members and friends, they still attributed their survival more often to their religious faith. In their analysis of these data, Elliott and Pais conclude, "Among blacks in the region, religious faith seems to be part of the communal glue that individuals and families use to cement social relationships and to ensure the emotional support that such relationships provide. So even when helping one another to cope, African Americans from the area are likely to report that it is God that has made this type of network assistance possible, not family or friends themselves. . . . These patterns suggest that in the regional 'black' model, faith is at the interpretive forefront, making all things possible."[57] This result is not surprising, considering that entire families and extended family networks in black communities were displaced. For African Americans abandoned for five days at the Convention Center or the Superdome, family members could offer emotional support, but not much in terms of material help. This is where organized churches played a key role.

Historically, Christian African Americans refer to their churches as "church homes" or "church families."[58] Their fellow church members often constitute major parts of their support systems. I have shown that church family members will often come to support a family through the death of a loved one.[59] Funerals are one of the most important rites of passage in African American culture. This was particularly true of New Orleans and other parts of Louisiana where the ritual of the jazz funeral was often practiced. These funerals provided a paradoxical combination of sadness at the loss of a deceased family member and celebration of the life of their loved one and their "homegoing" to heaven. Sadly, many African American families who were survivors of Katrina have not had the comfort of this church support or the familiar ritual of the funeral.

Given these realities, the trauma associated with Katrina survivors' and family members' inability to locate or identify their departed relatives and give them a "proper" funeral becomes even more poignant. Priscilla Dass-Brailsford described the height of cultural insensitivity in the aftermath of Katrina in which emergency responders were told, "'Ignore the dead. . . . We want the living.' The comment struck Dass-Brailsford as deeply insensitive to the strong kinship ties and religious values among African Americans in the Deep South. . . . 'They were not prepared to ignore their dead,' she said. 'In fact, they could not continue living until their dead had been accounted for and respectfully put to rest.'"[60] Many African American families have since had memorial services that have allowed some closure to their grief and loss. This is further testimony to the survival function of religion and spirituality in the African American community.

Katrina, finally, has had far-reaching implications for African Americans who see the church as a kind of home. Church families were scattered across the country, and numerous "church homes" of African Americans in the Gulf region were destroyed by Katrina. In many areas, a major cultural institution was lost.

Andrew Billingsley and Patricia Motes, family researchers, have studied the impact of the destruction and loss of black churches in the Gulf Coast communities most affected by Katrina, such as New Orleans and Mississippi. They also explored the experiences of churches in areas that provided shelter for large numbers of African American Katrina survivors in Houston, Texas; Memphis, Tennessee; and Columbia, South Carolina. Their research findings concluded that "before Hurricane Katrina, African American churches in the affected areas were prominent and functional features of community life. The destruction of these communities, including numerous churches and church holdings, such as community centers [and] housing developments . . . was rampant. Church leaders and church members were displaced physically and emotionally. Communities received support from other church congregations, across racial and denominational lines."[61] Billingsley and Motes also found evidence of the resilience of these churches and their members: "Church communities are providing financial and other tangible support, holding rallies, sharing pulpits, donating the use of church buildings, and helping to rebuild sanctuaries. Many community members expressed a renewal of community spirit and corresponding pride. Indicators of resilience and faith are evident despite enormous death and suffering. . . . And church leaders envision a return of the power and presence of the African American church in these devastated areas."[62]

Many African American families, displaced and spread throughout this country, have shown resilience in their attempts to reconnect with and rebuild their extended family networks. Extended families have opened their homes to large numbers of family members and have pooled resources in order to survive. Katrina destroyed many of the very old, poor African American communities in New Orleans, the rest of Louisiana, Mississippi, and Alabama, where family members had lived for generations. These areas had a unique culture composed of tight-knit networks of blood (grandparents, aunts, uncles, cousins, parents, siblings, etc.) as well as nonblood relatives (godparents, neighbors, "church family," and community members).[63] In general, the media failed to recognize that many victims' homes had been in their families for generations and were among the few possessions that they owned.[64] Instead, much of the media coverage after Hurricane Katrina adopted a "blame the victim" posture and passed judgment on these families for not evacuating before the storm.[65] Lost in the media coverage was the determination and resilience of many of these survivors, particularly those who stayed behind to defend their homes or to care for elderly relatives who were unable to leave.

Conclusion

Because so many Americans—including members of media; federal, state and local government officials; first responders; and average citizens—are unwilling to accept the reality of discrimination (let alone the levels of racism in society), many of the potential lessons of Katrina have been lost.[66] In summary, this chapter has explored the tragedy of Hurricane Katrina as a catastrophic disaster that has led to psychological trauma for countless African American survivors. As I have written elsewhere, this psychological trauma was made worse by the racism, discriminatory classism, and lack of respect that they experienced before, during, and after the storm. This chapter stands in tribute to the strength of these survivors, and I hope that it empowers all of us to use our collective voices to speak out against the racism, discrimination, and poverty that Katrina brought to our collective consciousness. Only then can we honor the requests of the survivors that we "never forget."

Unfortunately, the mistrust created by these experiences of racism may inadvertently shape the reaction and response of the black community to future disasters.[67] Any natural disaster can be exacerbated by the trauma of racism, but manifestations of racism may be subtle and may easily be denied by others.[68] For example, it is essential that aid-givers in the midst of chaotic crisis interventions have the trust of disaster victims. After Katrina, there were many reports of insensitivity among some of the well-meaning first responders.[69] If these personnel are not well trained in cultural sensitivity and ignore or fail to recognize African Americans' anger about their experiences of racism, they risk being unable to build that necessary trust and face the possibility of retraumatizing victims. This vicious circle may lead to greater loss of life. There are often emotional consequences of such denial for African Americans.

One of the greatest lessons of Hurricane Katrina has been the need for partnerships between the disaster relief agencies and African American churches. These faith-based organizations are arguably among the most powerful institutions in many black communities, and they can provide help on a physical, emotional, and spiritual level. More generally, if we, as a society, fail to recognize how Katrina continues to shape the black experience in America and the broader psychological vulnerability of being black in the United States, we risk repeating these mistakes and their unacknowledged but not less dire consequences.

NOTES

1. Linda Burton, Donna-Marie Winn, Howard Stevenson, and Sherri Lawson Clark, "Working with African American Clients: Considering the "Homeplace" in Marriage and Family Therapy Practices," *Journal of Marital and Family Therapy* 30 (2004): 397–410.
2. bell hooks, *Yearning: Race, Gender, and Cultural Politics* (Boston: South End Press, 1990), 42.
3. The African American survivors of Katrina lost more than their physical homes. Nancy Boyd-Franklin, "Working with African Americans and Trauma: Lessons for

Clinicians from Hurricane Katrina," in *Re-visioning Family Therapy: Race, Culture, and Gender in Clinical Practice*, ed. Monica McGoldrick and Kenneth V. Hardy, 2nd ed., 344–355 (New York: Guilford Press, 2009). Although individuals of all ethnic and racial groups may search for a sense of "home," this concept has a profound psychological meaning for African Americans, given their history of slavery, the diaspora, and the legacy of discrimination, segregation, and racism that have affected the lives of generations of African Americans. Nancy Boyd-Franklin, *Black Families in Therapy: Understanding the African American Experience*, 2nd ed. (New York: Guilford Press, 2003); Burton et al., "Working with African American Clients"; hooks, *Yearning*. The multigenerational cultural memory of African Americans, kept alive through the oral tradition of storytelling, reminds us that we were forcibly removed from our homes in Africa and transported under horrible conditions to slavery in America. In response to this catastrophic trauma, African Americans developed physical, spiritual, psychological, and emotional survival skills that foster multigenerational resilience. Boyd-Franklin, "Working with African Americans and Trauma." One survival skill is the development of a "home" or "homeplace." When media commentators questioned why so many African Americans had not evacuated their homes during Hurricane Katrina, they missed the obvious—many of these poor, New Orleans residents did not own cars or did not have the funds to stay in a hotel out of the pathway of the hurricane. Michael Eric Dyson, *Come Hell or High Water* (New York: Basic Civitas, 2006); David Troutt, *After the Storm: Black Intellectuals Explore the Meaning of Hurricane Katrina* (New York: New Press, 2006).

4. Government agencies, including the Federal Emergency Management Agency, have often focused their attention on helping survivors to find new homes. While this is an important and necessary part of recovery, it is not enough to heal the "soul wound" or psychological trauma created by the loss of one's homeplace. Boyd-Franklin, "Working with African Americans and Trauma."

5. Dyson, *Come Hell or High Water*; J. R. Elliott and J. Pais, "Race, Class, and Hurricane Katrina: Social Differences in Human Responses to Disaster," *Social Science Research* 35 (2006): 295–321; Troutt, *After the Storm*.

6. Boyd-Franklin, "Working with African Americans and Trauma"; Priscilla Dass-Brailsford, "Eye Witness Report: Ignore the Dead; We Want the Living! Helping after the Storm," *Communique* (March 2006): vi–viii; Dyson, *Come Hell or High Water*; Troutt, *After the Storm*.

7. Dyson, *Come Hell or High Water*; Troutt, *After the Storm*.

8. Tania Ralli, "Who's a Looter?: In Storm's Aftermath, Pictures Pick Up a Different Kind of Tempest," *New York Times*, September 5, 2005, http://www.nytimes.com/2005/09/05/business/05caption.html (accessed October 10, 2005).

9. Dyson, *Come Hell or High Water*; Troutt, *After the Storm*.

10. Samuel R. Sommers, Evan P. Apfelbaum, Kristin Dukes, Negin Toosi, and Elsie J. Wang, "Race and Media Coverage of Hurricane Katrina: Analysis, Implications, and Future Research Questions," *Analyses of Social Issues and Public Policy* 6, no. 1 (2006): 39–55.

11. Geoffrey Nunberg, "When Words Break Down," Nunberg's Web page, September 8, 2005, http://people.ischool.berkeley.edu/~nunberg/looting.html (accessed October 10, 2005).

12. Sommers et al., "Race and Media Coverage of Hurricane Katrina," 41.

13. Ibid.

14. Ibid.

15. Ibid.

16. Entman and Rojecki quoted in ibid., 45.

17. Kristin Henkel, John F. Dovidio, and Samuel L. Gaertner, "Institutional Discrimination, Individual Racism, and Hurricane Katrina," *Analyses of Social Issues and Public Policy* 6, no. 1 (2006): 99–124.

18. Ibid.

19. Aaron Sharockman, "Neighboring Town Denied Evacuees," *St. Petersburg Times*, September 17, 2005, 1.

20. Boyd-Franklin, "Working with African Americans and Trauma"; Dyson, *Come Hell or High Water*; Troutt, *After the Storm*.

21. Boyd-Franklin, *Black Families in Therapy*. Poll results mentioned in this paragraph are from CNN, "Reaction to Katrina Split along Racial Lines," CNN.com, September 13, 2005, http://www.cnn.com/2005/12/katrina.race.poll/index.html.

22. Robert T. Carter, "Racism and Psychological and Emotional Injury: Recognizing and Assessing Race-Based Traumatic Stress," *Counseling Psychologist* 35, no. 1 (2007): 13–105; Rodney Clark, Norman B. Anderson, Vanessa R. Clark, and David R. Williams, "Racism as a Stressor for African Americans: A Biopsychosocial Model," *American Psychologist* 54 (1999): 805–816; Shawn O. Utsey, Mark H. Chae, Christa F. Brown, and Deborah Kelly, "Effect of Ethnic Group Membership on Ethnic Identity, Race-Related Stress, and Quality of Life," *Cultural Diversity and Ethnic Minority Psychology* 8 (2002): 366–377.

23. CNN, "Reaction to Katrina Split along Racial Lines."

24. Carter, "Racism and Psychological and Emotional Injury"; Anderson James Franklin, Nancy Boyd-Franklin, and Shalonda Kelly, "Racism and Invisibility: Race-Related Stress, Emotional Abuse, and Psychological Trauma for People of Color," *Journal of Emotional Abuse* 6, no. 2/3 (2006): 9–30.

25. Boyd-Franklin, "Working with African Americans and Trauma"; CNN, "Reaction to Katrina Split along Racial Lines."

26. Peggy McIntosh, "White Privilege: Unpacking the Invisible Knapsack," in *Re-visioning Family Therapy*, ed. Monica McGoldrick and Kenneth V. Hardy, 2nd ed., 147–152 (New York: Guilford Press, 2009).

27. Franklin, Boyd-Franklin, and Kelly, "Racism and Invisibility"; Lisa Blitz and Mary Pender Greene, eds., *Racism and Racial Identity: Reflections on Urban Practice in Mental Health and Social Services* (Binghamton, N.Y.: Haworth Press, 2006); James Jones, *Prejudice and Racism*, 2nd ed. (New York: McGraw-Hill, 1997).

28. Dyson, *Come Hell or High Water*; Janet B. Ruscher, "Stranded by Katrina: Past and Present," *Analyses of Social Issues and Public Policy* 6, no. 1 (2006): 33–38; Troutt, *After the Storm*.

29. Shelly P. Harrell, "A Multidimensional Conceptualization of Racism-Related Stress: Implications for the Well-Being of People of Color," *American Journal of Orthopsychiatry* 70 (2000): 42–57.

30. Dyson, *Come Hell or High Water*; Troutt, *After the Storm*.

31. Dyson, *Come Hell or High Water*.

32. Henkel, Dovidio, and Gaertner, "Institutional Discrimination, Individual Racism, and Hurricane Katrina," 101.

33. Ibid.

34. Ibid., 102.

35. Dyson, *Come Hell or High Water*; Ruscher, "Stranded by Katrina: Past and Present"; Troutt, *After the Storm*.

36. Harrell, "A Multidimensional Conceptualization of Racism-Related Stress." Concerning transgenerational transmission, see also Franklin, Boyd-Franklin, and Kelly, "Racism and Invisibility." Concerning microaggressions, see also Anderson James Franklin, *From Brotherhood to Manhood: How Black Men Rescue Their Relationships and Dreams from the Invisibility Syndrome* (Hoboken, N.J.: John Wiley, 2004); Chester Pierce, "Stress Analogs of Racism and Sexism: Terrorism, Torture, and Disaster," in *Mental Health, Racism, and Sexism*, ed. Charles Willie, Patricia Perri Reiker, Bernard M. Kramer, and Bertram S. Brown, 277–293 (Pittsburgh: University of Pittsburgh Press, 1995).

37. Boyd-Franklin, *Black Families in Therapy*.

38. Henkel, Dovidio, and Gaertner, "Institutional Discrimination, Individual Racism, and Hurricane Katrina."

39. Hugh F. Butts has argued that the *Diagnostic and Statistical Manual of Mental Disorders* (DSM–IV-TR) (American Psychological Association, 2000) does not discuss racism as a trauma despite the fact that it can be extreme and catastrophic. Never was this more apparent than during Hurricane Katrina. See Hugh F. Butts, "The Black Mask of Humanity: Racial/Ethnic Discrimination and Post-Traumatic Stress Disorder," *Journal of the American Academy of Psychiatry and Law* 30 (2002): 336–339.

40. Carter, "Racism and Psychological and Emotional Injury"; Franklin, Boyd-Franklin, and Kelly, "Racism and Invisibility"; Blitz and Pender Greene, *Racism and Racial Identity*; Clark et al., "Racism as a Stressor for African Americans"; Utsey et al., "Effect of Ethnic Group Membership on Ethnic Identity."

41. Elliott and Pais, "Race, Class, and Hurricane Katrina."

42. Dyson, *Come Hell or High Water*; Troutt, *After the Storm*.

43. Reported in "Levels of Serious Mental Illness in Katrina Survivors Doubled," *Science Daily*, August 29, 2006, http://www.sciencedaily.com/releases/2006/08/060828211642.htm.

44. Ibid.

45. Kaiser Family Foundation, "Major House-to-House Survey Finds New Orleans Area Residents Hit Hard by Katrina and Struggling with Serious Life Challenges," May 10, 2007, http://www.kff.org/kaiserpolls/pomr051007nr.cfm.

46. Ibid., 2–3.

47. Ruscher, "Stranded by Katrina," 33.

48. Ibid.

49. BBSNEWS, "Hurricane Katrina Is Not Over: Eighteen Months after Katrina," February 27, 2007; http://bbsnews.net/article.php/2007022723050030I.

50. Ibid., 1.

51. Ibid.

52. Ibid.

53. Ruscher, "Stranded by Katrina."

54. Ibid.

55. Boyd-Franklin, *Black Families in Therapy*.

56. Robert J. Taylor, Jacqueline Mattis, and Linda M. Chatters, "Subjective Religiosity among African Americans: A Synthesis of Findings from Five National Samples," *Journal of Black Psychology* 25 (1999): 524–543.

57. Elliott and Pais, "Race, Class, and Hurricane Katrina," 315.

58. There is a tremendous amount of diversity in the African American community in terms of spirituality and religion—and particular church organizations have played a role in building resilience in the face of crisis. Many African Americans are not church-involved but have a strong spiritual belief in God and turn to prayer in times of trouble. In addition, many religious denominations are represented in African American communities: Baptist, Methodist, AME, Catholic, Episcopalian, Presbyterian, Lutheran, Pentecostal, Church of God in Christ, Jehovah's Witnesses, and Seventh Day Adventists. Many African Americans are also members of non-Christian groups such as the Nation of Islam and Sunni Muslim groups. A small number practice African religions. Boyd-Franklin, *Black Families in Therapy*.

59. Boyd-Franklin, "Working with African Americans and Trauma."

60. Dass-Brailsford quoted in B. M. Law, "The Hard Work of Healing: Katrina's Cultural Lessons," *APA Monitor on Psychology* 9 (October 27, 2006): 40.

61. Andrew Billingsley and Patricia Motes, "The Role of the African American Church in Promoting Post-catastrophe Resilience," University of South Carolina, Hurricane Katrina Crisis, http://www.sc.edu/katrinacrisis/billingsley_motes.shtml.

62. Ibid, 2.

63. Boyd-Franklin, *Black Families in Therapy*.

64. Boyd-Franklin, "Working with African Americans and Trauma."

65. Jaime L. Napier, Anesu N. Mandisodza, and Susan M. Anderson, and John Jost, "System Justification in Responding to the Poor and Displaced in the Aftermath of Hurricane Katrina," *Analyses of Social Issues and Public Policy* 6, no. 1 (2006): 57–73.

66. Boyd-Franklin, "Working with African Americans and Trauma"; CNN, "Reaction to Katrina Split along Racial Lines"; Dyson, *Come Hell or High Water*; Troutt, *After the Storm*.

67. Henkel, Dovidio, and Gaertner, "Institutional Discrimination, Individual Racism, and Hurricane Katrina."

68. Blitz and Pender Greene, *Racism and Racial Identity*; Carter, "Racism and Psychological and Emotional Injury"; Franklin, Boyd-Franklin, and Kelly, "Racism and Invisibility."

69. Dass-Brailsford, "Eye Witness Report."

8

The Haunted Houses
of New Orleans

Gothic Homelessness and
African American Experience

EVIE SHOCKLEY

Among the most potent images of post–Hurricane Katrina New Orleans are those depicting the wind-wrecked, water-ravaged, molding, abandoned houses. Neighborhoods nearest the levee breaches, like the predominantly African American Lower Ninth Ward, were filled with street after street of such structures after the storm. Even more disturbing, perhaps, are pictures of ragged lots that once held homes but were left empty when storm and floodwaters washed away everything except the concrete blocks upon which the buildings used to sit—the white, irregularly spaced rectangles unnervingly calling to mind tombstones. Photographs of individual houses tilting wildly at impossible angles or sitting on top of cars, of whole rows of clearly uninhabitable dwellings tagged with spray-painted body counts, speak eloquently to the destruction of lives and property.

They testify as well as to the massive numbers of residents who found themselves suddenly displaced; the then-acting director of the Federal Emergency Management Agency estimated in October 2005 that between four hundred thousand and six hundred thousand people had been left homeless by the disaster.[1] As the waters receded, the absence of former New Orleans residents became a presence in itself: an eerie specter hovering over the silent, empty streets of areas like the Lower Ninth Ward, Tremé, and Gentilly. Though some were able to return—and new populations arrived, drawn by the opportunities the massive rebuilding effort promised—even two years later, in 2007, the population of the city remained at only 60 percent of its pre-Katrina number; as of 2009, that figure had crept up to 76.4 percent.[2] Headlines a year and more afterward described New Orleans as "haunted" by Katrina, and references to the city and neighborhoods like the Lower Ninth as "ghost towns" proliferated.[3] The language of the gothic—of terrors and horrors, of inescapable nightmares and life-in-death—offered an effective, emotionally accurate way to communicate the chilling experience of returning to and attempting to survive in this place that so many people had called home.

Before the Deluge: Domestic Ideology and the Concept of Home

But the homes of some residents of New Orleans had been haunted houses long before Katrina came to town. The simple, small, worn, but perfectly livable houses of African Americans living in the Lower Ninth and other poor neighborhoods have perhaps always been populated by ghosts: among others, the *absent presence* of racist stereotypes that imagine those houses not as homes, but as places where no one could "really" live—in effect, as tombs. One of these ghosts raised its horrible head in the Houston Astrodome, to which thousands of Katrina survivors—survivors not simply of the storm, but also of the horrors of the New Orleans Superdome and Convention Center—were finally evacuated after days of waiting. It took the form of a remark made by former First Lady Barbara Bush, who was interviewed during a visit to the stadium. Pictures and reports set the scene: the predominantly black survivors huddled over their meager possessions on narrow cots arranged by Red Cross volunteers in long rows and columns across the Astrodome floor. John Nichols, writing for *The Nation*, emphasized the relentless sensory assault of conditions there: "cots crammed side-by-side in a huge stadium where the lights never go out and the sound of sobbing children never completely ceases."[4] In response to a question about her exchanges with the people she was meeting, Bush comments, "What I'm hearing, which is sort of scary, is they all want to stay in Texas. Everyone is so overwhelmed by the hospitality. And so many of the people in the arena here, you know, were underprivileged anyway, so this, this is working very well for them."[5]

This chilling observation (or "blindness" might be the better word), accompanied by an audible chuckle, was widely covered by the press and provoked quite an outcry against Bush's thoughtlessness. Most of the people she met that day were indeed among New Orleans's most financially impoverished—as we know from Mia Bay's chapter, they were those whose "stubborn" insistence on "riding it out" was deeply informed by the practical calculations indicating that they simply could not afford to evacuate themselves. But to suggest that they were better off receiving disaster relief in the Astrodome than they were prior to Katrina is more than insensitive; it is to imagine them as having already been, in effect, *homeless*.

This way of thinking is not unique to Bush; rather, it is characteristic of an ideology that began in the late eighteenth century in England, accompanying the rise of the English middle classes and helping those groups to consolidate their growing political power. "Domestic ideology" not only romanticized and naturalized a newly developing conception of how homes and families should "properly" be organized, but it proposed individual homes and families as models for larger social systems—including the nation, with its "domestic borders" and "national family." As the housing and familial arrangements of the emerging middle classes shifted in response to the economic pressures and opportunities of the Industrial Revolution, a way of thinking (and a corresponding rhetoric) that tended to reify and justify those arrangements also surfaced.

The single-family residence, separated spatially from the workplace and business districts generally, became the archetype for "home, sweet home," and the nuclear family, composed of a heterosexual, married couple and their children, became not just common but also normative in the prescriptive sense. This ideology, in other words, posited a very class-based set of social arrangements as the norm in order to vilify (and obtain power over/from) the people of the working classes and the members of the aristocracy. The former were deemed "vulgar" and the latter "decadent" for their refusal (read: financial inability or lack of sociopolitical incentives) to conform their lives to the Puritan standards of thrift, modesty, and purity vaunted by the middle classes as the only decent and respectable way to live. Conformance, however—or the *performance* of conformance—was deemed a sign of virtue that identified those in the middle classes to one another and purportedly showed them to be the proper people to hold political power in England.[6] The way they would exercise that power was also determined with reference to this ideology. The nation was "home" to a geopolitically organized "family," and by this logic, from the proper organization of an individual family and its home one could elucidate the best ways of managing the domestic (and imperial) affairs of the nation.

Because domestic ideology prescribes and privileges the construction of "normal" homes and families around hierarchical principles and "inherent" social roles, its extension into the public sociopolitical realm only magnifies the ideology's discriminatory impact. For example, domestic ideology encourages us to assume that "the woman's place is within the home," that "the man is the head of the household," and that "father knows best" what his children need. Such axioms underwrite and perpetuate dramatic inequities even among those who are ostensibly the ideology's beneficiaries—limiting, for instance, the middle-class Victorian Englishwoman's ability to become a wage earner and live independently of a father or husband. The effects of these axioms are all the more pernicious among individuals and groups upon whom the ideology is imposed—such as the "childlike" people of color whose well-being was said to require the paternalistic British imperial rule.

Domestic ideology thus has deep ties to the colonial enterprise and, likewise, to the attitudes that justified the enslavement of Africans in the "New World." People who did not live in "homes" on the British model might well not be "people" at all, but subhuman creatures provided on the earth, like horses and cattle, for the benefit of those who could profit from them—or, more generously, such uncivilized groups needed the firm hand of the white man to "raise" them from their "primitive" state. In this way, age and class hierarchies underwriting the social roles within the white, middle-class family were mapped onto racist socioeconomic structures in Britain's colonial empire and, after a time, in the United States, which appeared to have imported domestic ideology along with other products from the "mother country."[7] Anglo-American constructions of African "homelessness" connect in painfully ironic ways with the literal, collective homelessness of Africans in America and their descendents. Survivors of the Middle Passage found themselves a part of the most massive involuntary displacement of human beings in our history—a violent, forced migration carried out purposefully so as to prevent the retention of kinship groups, languages, or cultural practices that might have enabled black people to (re)create a home for themselves in the United States. The nearly four centuries of violent, racist disregard for black humanity on what is now U.S. territory and the long-standing, ongoing history of blacks' physical and cultural displacement here combine to create a kind of *social terror* that circulates consistently through African American culture. I have called this social terror "gothic homelessness,"[8] and I argue here that gothic homelessness has made the Katrina disaster a particularly harrowing experience for African Americans—and not only those from New Orleans.

Gothic Homelessness and Social Terror

Barbara Bush's comment, as one element of that Katrina experience, raises the specter of gothic homelessness because it exposes the continuing currency of the stereotype of African American residences as being less than "homes"—not really *domestic* spaces. If domestic ideology asks us to think in terms of a private/public divide, with the "home" as a kind of safe haven from the dangers, diseases, and degradation of the streets (or the workplace, or foreign soil—or whatever might be placed in opposition to the domestic refuge), African Americans have been doubly denied participation in this social configuration. On one hand, African American dwellings have been made permeable (by law or lawlessness) to Ku Klux Klan posses, police invasion, state welfare agencies, and unchecked crime, among other things, that disturb one's privacy and the quiet enjoyment of one's residence. On the other hand, white Americans have constructed images of African Americans, especially poor and working-class African Americans, as choosing to live in squalor—as a result of a "natural" tendency toward uncleanliness, laziness, or other vices that leave no time for keeping house—and thus lacking the domesticity that marks one as virtuous, industrious, and (therefore) deserving of the full rights and privileges of citizenship in a modern nation. The disempowerment of black people that is built into the structure of most U.S. political and economic institutions is not acknowledged as a contributing, sometimes determining, factor in the state of African Americans' domestic lives. Nevertheless, African Americans' "standard" domesticity is offered as a justification for denying them the privileges and opportunities that would afford them a real choice about whether and how to embrace ideologically dominant constructions of domesticity.

The circularity of domestic ideology's logic as applied to African Americans—which contributes significantly to policies and practices that sharply delimit opportunities for black upward social mobility—constitutes a conceptual entrapment that is made manifest in de jure and de facto segregation in education, employment, and, of course, housing. For African Americans, aware of their collective assignment to the lowest reaches of U.S. society, the effort to make a better life for themselves and their families can be like trying to escape from a social dungeon, a dark and endless maze whose doors often turn out to be locked from the outside. This state of affairs combines with the ongoing threat of more immediate violence to produce a social terror that is palpable in African American culture. One of the sites in which this social terror is made manifest is African American literature; indeed, I derived the term "gothic homelessness" as a name for this African American experience of social terror from African American writers' long practice of using the gothic genre's tropes and conventions to inscribe in literature this element of our experience. Thus the language of the gothic that, as I noted in the opening of this chapter, has been repeatedly invoked to describe the literal homelessness evident in post-Katrina New Orleans, is also the language that African American literature employs to communicate the terror of forms of homelessness that include, but exceed, having no place to live. This confluence is as apt historically as it is telling with regard to the Katrina context today.

The history of the gothic genre is thus worth exploring here, briefly, as a foundation for understanding its present usefulness in thinking about New Orleans's haunted houses. The gothic genre had its origins in the English literary tradition more than two hundred years ago, when Harold Walpole's *The Castle of Otranto* gained an enthusiastic audience for its tale of a royal family's doom, and the genre continues to be popular with writers (and now filmmakers) and audiences in the twenty-first century. The genre's fundamental characteristic is that it is designed to communicate to readers or viewers feelings of intense terror or horror. Far from being purely punitive, this goal recognizes the pleasure that such feelings can bring when safely contained within the pages of a book or the frames of a movie—by analogy, we might think of the mix of excitement and anxiety (the "thrills") that a roller-coaster ride generates. Equally important, the gothic is intended to produce a catharsis in its audience: to articulate its readers' fears in a form that allows them to be resolved—in narrative, if not in life. Exemplars of the gothic genre include such well-known horror stories as Mary Shelley's *Frankenstein*, Bram Stoker's *Dracula*, and

Alfred Hitchcock's *Psycho*, as well as tales of sublime terror ranging from *The Mysteries of Udolpho* (Ann Radcliffe's eighteenth-century best seller) to Charlotte Brontë's *Jane Eyre* to Toni Morrison's *Beloved*. Certain figures, settings, tones, and plot devices that early gothic texts like Walpole's and Radcliffe's novels used to create the effect of terror in readers have appeared in subsequent works so frequently as to become conventional. Some things that readers have come to expect from the genre are depictions of restless ghosts, dark and labyrinthine dungeons, eerie doppelgängers, grotesque monsters, chilling murders, cold-blooded cruelty, blood-curdling screams, and unending nightmares—all rendered in language carefully chosen to heighten the audience's emotions. As many of these examples indicate, the gothic is a genre of the *fantastic*, which is to say that it characteristically includes events that are supernatural, incredible, or, at the very least, bizarre, and it often asks audiences to accept as fact occurrences that would not be considered possible in ordinarily rational terms.

Some gothic conventions that are particularly relevant for my purpose here illuminate the cultural significance of the family and the home as loci of important social anxieties. The plots of early gothic novels typically involved issues of family lineage and legacy, in which rightful heirs were restored to their families and inheritances or heroines of dubious background were ultimately found to be of noble birth and therefore proper candidates for marriage to young, aristocratic men. Ghosts and other supernatural phenomena were often the vehicles through which past wrongs were righted in order to reaffirm the legitimacy of a family; fantastic events intervened to ensure that all interlopers were expunged and only those who belonged in the "house" remained inside it at the novel's close. An older woman who was inexplicably and eerily similar to a young orphan would be revealed to be her double's long-lost mother, for instance; or the ruins of a family's castle would contain the evidence of a dastardly plot to disinherit a nobleman's son, just in time to prevent it from being achieved. This preoccupation with home and family among early British gothic novelists was no coincidence. The heyday of those classic gothic works was between 1764 (when *Otranto* was published) and about 1830—virtually the same period in which the emerging middle classes of England were developing domestic ideology as a means of legitimating their claims to power. The right to govern England was at stake, and by 1832, when the Reform Act was passed giving the franchise to a much wider range of voters and shifting the balance of power in Parliament to the House of Commons, the tide had turned. Domesticity, the stronghold of the middle classes, had become in many respects a quintessential sign of Englishness, both culturally and politically. Any threat to domesticity, or to the ideology of domesticity, had serious ramifications and produced deep—gothic—anxieties. The home was constructed as a haven, a place where the family is safe; to fulfill that function, it had to be, or be made to seem, invulnerable.

The gothic genre, then, was fertile literary territory for African American authors, whose domestic concerns have been consistently shaped by the vulnerability of the "homeless." Those concerns have included everything from the loss of the original African home(land) to the breaking up of families for sale under slavery to the exclusion of black people from the American national "family" (those possessing the rights and privileges of citizenship that protect one, for example, from murder, rape, and theft) —all sources of almost unimaginable terror and horror. Indeed, one of the things that further contributed to the serviceability of the gothic for African American writers' purposes was the element of the fantastic the genre incorporates. The reality of black experience in the United States has often been so excessive, so impossibly horrific, that it is more surreal than real. Since as early as the 1845 publication of the *Narrative of the Life of Frederick Douglass*, African American writers have turned to a genre in which the unbelievable occurs as a matter of course in order to convey unbelievably frightening conditions of existence.

After Katrina: Outside the National Home

The lens of gothic homelessness, then, allows us to see not simply the *fact* of Katrina's devastation of a once majority-black city but also the *social meaning* of that loss for African Americans—individually and collectively, within the "Katrina diaspora" and beyond it.[9] If, for example, the emotional response of African Americans born and raised elsewhere in the United States has seemed inapposite to their geographical and material distance from the epicenter of the disaster's damage, identifying the relationship of forced migration and displacement to gothic homelessness can help explain its intensity. The Middle Passage—that terrifying journey across the Atlantic in the dark, underwater nightmare that the hold of the slave ships constituted—might be seen as the "originary" gothic horror; it meant the irreversible loss of home for the millions of people unfortunate enough to begin it. This journey ended in death or permanent expatriation, and just as surely meant the loss of family bonds, for even in the absence of physical separation, the refusal of American law and custom to recognize familial relationships among the enslaved rendered those relationships practically (if not emotionally) meaningless.[10] Further, because African cultural practices (including the use of indigenous languages and performance of religious rituals) were sometimes outlawed, often forbidden, and otherwise ruptured by the careful dispersal of the various ethnic groups from which Africans were drawn into slavery, within one or two generations the homeland was effectively lost to memory as well.

African Americans from most parts of the U.S. South underwent a second major upheaval during the early twentieth-century period known as the Great Migration, when the lure of northern industrial jobs and the need to escape de facto slavery under the southern sharecropping system combined to draw more than a million out of the region and into cities like Chicago, Pittsburgh, Detroit, and New York. It was in New Orleans, by contrast, where black people not only found themselves able to retain a number of African cultural practices, such as drumming, that were illegal elsewhere but also chose to stay, generation upon generation, in favor of going to climates that were colder (in both senses of the word). The ways that French and Spanish colonies managed slavery differed from the British approaches that had set the tone elsewhere in the United States. Insofar as French and Spanish attitudes that helped to shape New Orleans culture were less invested in suppressing and erasing African influences, those influences became integral to the way of life in that city.[11] As Richard Mizelle's chapter reminds us, African Americans could look to New Orleans for speech patterns, cuisine, rituals, philosophies, and, significantly, music that were as close as we might get to the unknowable African past. One did not have to be from New Orleans to value what it represented for African American culture.

Thus, the loss of New Orleans as a space of considerable African American cultural continuity was a signal catastrophe for African Americans across the country, because it magnified the extent of our collective homelessness. Had the Katrina disaster been primarily a testament to the forces of nature unleashed on a human habitat, this loss would have been painful enough. But instead, the greatest material damage—the flooding that turned a temporary evacuation into a permanent dislocation for so many New Orleanians—resulted from the apparent indifference of federal, state, and local governments to the threat hurricanes had increasingly posed to the levee system protecting the city. To this injury was added the insultingly—fatally—slow government efforts to rescue and provide aid to the people trapped in New Orleans after the storm without the food, water, and medical care they needed. The disaster provided horrifying evidence of the relative unimportance of the residents and the city itself to this nation and even the state of Louisiana—at least as represented by governmental policies and actions. Bereft of strong, direct connections to our places of origin on the African continent, African Americans were cruelly reminded during the aftermath of Katrina that our condition of gothic homelessness continues to this day because we have not yet, in the United States's more than 230-year history, been accepted and treated as full citizens, as members of the "national family."

It always bears repeating that the U.S. Constitution was originally drafted and ratified to enshrine inequality, rather than to abolish it. Citizenship, for human beings who were legally counted as three-fifths of a person in determining a state's congressional representation, could only be a remote dream. And though by 1964, the combined force of the Fourteenth, Fifteenth, Nineteenth, and Twenty-fourth Amendments had ensured that all people—including the descendents (men and women) of Africans and the enslaved—had the fundamental citizen's right of voting, the extent of African Americans' citizenship was called seriously into question by various governmental responses to the predominantly black New Orleanians who remained there as the floodwaters rose. If citizenship is the status of *belonging* within the nation's domestic boundaries, this status was denied to New Orleanians who were prevented from leaving the city by Jefferson Parish police.[12] The Crescent City Connection, a bridge with entrance ramps virtually at the doors of the New Orleans Convention Center, crosses over the Mississippi River and touches down in the town of Gretna, in Louisiana's Jefferson Parish. It was at no point rendered impassable by the storm or subsequent flooding. But the Gretna police chief cut off this route to the resources New Orleanians so desperately needed. He ordered his officers to line up across the bridge and deny passage to the eight hundred or so survivors who had walked the three sweltering miles from the Convention Center to a place where they believed they would receive help. The police officers shot their guns over the heads of the advancing group, which was described in a news report as "overwhelmingly black," reinforcing the physical barrier of their linked bodies with the threat of violent force. Karen Carter, a Louisiana state representative for New Orleans, commented on this telling moment in Spike Lee's documentary *When the Levees Broke*: "Well, I thought that I lived in America until shortly after Katrina, and the Crescent City Connection was blocked off from people being able to walk freely on United States soil. . . . It was unjust, it was inhumane, and unacceptable."[13] Carter's comment highlights the way racist stereotypes about African Americans translated into a tangible boundary to "protect" the citizens from the "thugs," as the exhausted and traumatized New Orleanians were called, who apparently did not belong within the state and national perimeters.[14]

This armed, uniformed, state-ordered boundary, insofar as it operated to redefine the geopolitical contours of the nation, recalls the Border Patrol that divides the United States from Mexico. It constituted a similarly potent symbol of the line between those who possess the full rights and privileges of U.S. citizenship and those who do not—a symbol of discriminatory treatment that was not created, but only made visible, by the crisis. African Americans, who have only enjoyed the *appearance* of full citizenship for a few decades, are vitally aware of the extent to which we have functioned through most of this nation's history as aliens in our native land; hence the African American community nationwide responded with outrage when the media reports began referring to the people evacuated at last from the Superdome and the Convention Center—and displaced New Orleanians generally—as "refugees."[15] Gralen B. Banks, director of security at the Hyatt Hotel adjacent to the New Orleans Convention Center, gave voice to this perspective in an interview with Spike Lee: "'Refugees?' . . . Damn, when the storm came in that blew away our citizenship, too? . . . What?

We wasn't American citizens anymore? . . . Refugees. I thought that was folks who didn't have a country."[16] Though some commentators made the valid point that "refugee" also means "simply 'one seeking refuge,'" most had to acknowledge that the term was most frequently employed for its political definition, referring to "a person crossing national boundaries because of persecution,"[17] and in response to the outrage many African Americans expressed, most media outlets refrained from using it in the Katrina context after the first few days.[18]

Ironically, of course, the very thing that made the political connotations of the term so offensive to African Americans also made it an apt term for describing the ostensible status of the impoverished New Orleanians who were the last to be evacuated from the city. To suggest that all those thousands of Americans were like "refugees," in the political sense, should have been a slap in the face—not to the survivors, but to the federal government whose inept and/or indifferent response to the hurricane placed them in such dire straits that comparisons to displaced people of Haiti and Kosovo seemed warranted.[19] One might have wished that more African Americans had been careful not to imply, in their outrage, that there is something inherently shameful in the status of refugees, which—besides being false—is an implication not necessary to the argument that the Katrina survivors were being treated shamefully by the federal government and the media, too, at times. But this point should not obscure the additional bases of comparison between devastating post-Katrina conditions in New Orleans and the conditions of so-called Third World cities and even war zones, not to mention the painfully ironic similarities noted between the people of New Orleans and the people of Iraq as recipients of "aid" from the U.S. military—at gunpoint. In a nation that prides itself on protecting its citizens from the dangers and deprivations that others around the world must all too often suffer, New Orleanians have had to weather the storm, so to speak, outside of that shelter. If domestic ideology teaches that one's "home" is one's refuge, to be an African American "refugee" within the U.S. borders is to experience, yet again, gothic homelessness.

This exclusion from the shelter of citizenship has left the Katrina survivors exposed not only to danger but also to view. Ann Fabian's chapter draws attention to the relationship of the spectacle to gothic homelessness in perhaps its grimmest phase. Fabian's discussion of the dead bodies that were so memorably and disturbingly on display in the media coverage of Katrina juxtaposes their hypervisibility with the contrasting prohibition on media images of the remains of military personnel killed in Iraq. A Pentagon spokesperson said that the media ban was to demonstrate to the families of fallen soldiers that "[w]e respect and protect their privacy diligently."[20] The victims of Katrina and their families, on the other hand, had no privacy interests the media was bound to respect. As Nicole Fleetwood, a scholar of visual culture, writes in her analysis of the role of technology in "the Katrina event," "Visual media exposed bodies emoting, bodies suffering, bodies bloated and decaying, bodies—live and dead—as obstacles to be removed so that 'disaster capitalism' could begin its work of rebuilding what has been described as a dead city."[21] Fleetwood suggests persuasively that these were the bodies of the "living dead," in the eyes of the state, long before Katrina struck New Orleans. If so, then their sudden, disturbing, yet riveting visibility on televisions across the United States might be understood, from the perspective of the astonished white viewers, as a glimpse into the "tomb" to which this nation had consigned them. But to the poor and black survivors trapped in the ruins of their beloved hometown, the exposure of their grief, misery, and loss to curious, shocked, and even sympathetic spectators would constitute another predictable element of gothic homelessness.

The gruesome history of lynching in the United States, for example, foreshadows the aftermath of Katrina, for African Americans and others familiar with that aspect of our national past. From the post-Reconstruction era through the first decades of the twentieth century, white mobs thought nothing of forcing an African American out of his dwelling at any time of day or night and hanging, burning, or otherwise torturing him to death. These macabre events were far from covert; they were enacted by unmasked people, attended by white families as a type of social event, and reported in white and black newspapers.[22] Indeed, enough photographs of lynchings were taken (and frequently used in that era to decorate postcards) to fill a book: *Without Sanctuary: Lynching Photography in America*.[23] As the collection's title makes clear, African Americans were nowhere safe from the threat of this type of violence, least of all in their own homes. Moreover, the photographic display of dead black bodies constituted a second layer of violence to which African Americans were subject. The fact that accusations of rape, based on (and perpetuating) racist stereotypes of animalistic black hypersexuality, were frequently used to justify the murderous actions and attitudes of white communities only underscores the operation of domestic ideology in the construction of national acceptance of the practice of lynching. Domestic ideology participates similarly in shaping the acceptability of taking and publishing photographs of as-yet-unidentified drowning victims in New Orleans. The national exclusion that these published photographs symbolizes only reminds African Americans of how terrifyingly exposed to view, how gothically homeless we are.

This critique of media representations of Katrina, though necessary, has its limits. It is an unavoidable fact that by exposing the bodies of Katrina's dead and the suffering of its survivors, the media coverage also exposed the government's failures and created the impetus for faster, more efficient relief efforts by the government, as well as nongovernmental organizations, ad hoc groups, and individuals. Coverage seemed designed to create an outpouring of sympathy and philanthropy, yet even here the racial othering that perpetuates gothic homelessness comes into play. Arguably, the media template for reporting on

Katrina was developed in documenting the apparently endless misery to be found on the African continent and in other places around the globe where large numbers of people must bear with unbearable conditions. Such spectacles of abject black (and brown) suffering continue to be intricately related to efforts to raise awareness in people who might be able to intervene and relieve it. Yet, it must be acknowledged that without the television and radio broadcasts of images and firsthand accounts of the desperate conditions in New Orleans, which made people all over the United States and beyond witnesses to the government's failure to respond, help would have been even slower in arriving. Not only did these media reports spur the government to action—at last—but, according to Fleetwood, they also provided intelligence for the belated relief effort. In her discussion of the impact of technology in the context of Hurricane Katrina, she notes that the military relied on media reports to determine how best to distribute rescue and aid resources.[24]

It would be hard, then, to argue that the media did not play a critical role in the aftermath of Katrina. Nonetheless, the fact that news reports were needed to impress on the government that this degree of suffering was happening in America, signals—just as clearly as the disregard for the sufferers' privacy that some of the coverage entailed—that the citizenship of the predominantly black Katrina survivors is something less than the citizenship of U.S. soldiers and their families.[25] Additionally, the ways of thinking about African American bodies and lives that such media coverage promotes do not confine themselves to those channels that are most likely to help the African American objects of the curious (white) gaze. A prime example of this point can be found in the emergence, during the rebirth of New Orleans tourism, of "disaster tours." Charging anywhere from $35 to $50, tour companies began as early as December 2005 offering visitors to post-Katrina New Orleans, by the van- and bus-load, the opportunity to see firsthand the most devastated areas of the city and surrounding areas. The officials of at least one company indicated that they would donate a few dollars from each ticket to hurricane relief charities, and they and others have pointed to the awareness-raising and educational value of the tours.[26] Still, the tours are facilitating—for a profit—the framing of Katrina victims' lives as a spectacle for consumption by people who are more likely to spend the rest of their visit drinking hurricanes than cleaning up after them.[27]

Tourists are particularly interested in seeing the Lower Ninth Ward,[28] where they snap pictures through the windows of their vehicles as former residents of the area search for salvageable possessions, cut up fallen trees, and gut the houses in which they had lived for long years. Not all survivors are happy or comfortable with this type of attention. With their homes destroyed, they have no means of preserving their privacy as they grieve and work. One reporter noted that "[t]he more adventurous [tourists] treat the storm-battered homes like free museums, entering houses or yards for an intimate look at nature's fury."[29] While this disregard for privacy must be painful for any Katrina survivor, with regard to African Americans it resonates against a long history of spectacularization of black bodies and lives. Like other people of color from so-called primitive cultures, for centuries black people have been put on display for the "aesthetic contemplation, scientific analysis, and entertainment" of whites in Europe and North America. Often these living exhibitions of otherness were characterized and advertised as "ethnological"—that is, pseudoscientific and ostensibly educational.[30] For a relatively recent example, in 1906, a Pygmy man named Ota Benga was "put on display in the primate cage of the Bronx Zoo," where thousands of people came to gawk at him.[31] A letter to the editor of the *New York Times* highlighted the educational nature of the proceedings, which was apparently lost on the African American ministers who protested against the way Ota Benga was being treated: "It is a pity that Dr. Hornaday [the director of the zoo] does not introduce the system of short lectures or talks in connection with such exhibitions. This would emphasize the scientific character of the service, enhance immeasurably the usefulness of the Zoological Park to our public in general, and help our clergymen familiarize themselves with the scientific point of view so absolutely foreign to many of them."[32] The interest of whites in firsthand knowledge about unimaginable difference was recurrently seen to outweigh the interests of the exhibited people of color in their own privacy—not to mention their rights to mobility. I hope it is obvious that I am not *equating* the case of Ota Benga with the situation in New Orleans. Ota Benga was held captive, whereas the residents of the Ninth Ward are not forced to subject themselves to the tourist gaze (though to avoid it is to delay the work of recovery and return), as it is the physical devastation of the neighborhood that is of primary interest to the spectators. Nevertheless, the potential for profit, the quest for knowledge, *and* the voyeuristic consumption of fascinating spectacles are as intricately linked in the present case of Katrina "disaster tours" as in the historical examples of which Ota Benga is only one.[33] The effect of this history of racial spectacularization is to magnify the ghoulish, gothic aspect of disaster tourism for African Americans within and beyond the Lower Ninth.[34]

Indefinite Displacement

The Lower Ninth Ward, home to generations of African Americans, "lies in ruins": a haunted house.[35] Over the two years following the hurricane, in other parts of the city, including the recently developed neighborhoods of black professionals in New Orleans East, enough residents had, or have been provided, the resources necessary to rebuild and return home so that they have been able to create a look and feel of near normalcy. But the onetime residents of the Ninth Ward, though predominantly homeowners, have not been able to re-create the neighborhood's former homeyness. Too many have been unable to afford to get back from the various locations around the country where the belated evacuation stranded them.[36] Indeed, their ownership of homes on which they owed relatively little or nothing at all—homes that, in some cases, they had built with their own hands—was what made it possible for them to live comfortable lives on relatively little money.[37] Rents were low enough in pre-Katrina New Orleans that the same could be said of renters in the neighborhood. Without suggesting that the Lower Ninth was a paradise, we have to understand that the admittedly lower-income residents of the area did not see their lives as impoverished or their neighborhood as unsafe. As former resident Theodora Guilbeaux explained, "I never considered myself being poor. . . . I always thought I was average. Poor is when you can't afford to buy your baby Pampers or milk. You can't afford to put shoes on their feet. When you can take and hold down a job and you can have your children in parochial school, and you're paying $100 a week, that ain't poor. And that was what we were doing."[38] Despite their self-images as hard-working, family-oriented, culturally rich people, the African Americans of the Lower Ninth Ward have not been encouraged to return in any material way, by their insurance companies, the government, or their former employers. Barbara Bush's ghastly comment in the Astrodome illuminates the role of domestic ideology in the way this overwhelmingly black district of New Orleans is viewed by others.

Domestic ideology values fiscal conservatism and the ability to hold down a well-paying job, offering these characteristics—manifested in the ownership and maintenance of clean, well-appointed, spacious homes—as evidence of middle-class meritoriousness. By the same token, it explains poverty and the living conditions of the poor as the results of a refusal to work and, thus, as being fundamentally the fault of the poor.[39] This logic depends on a few rags-to-riches stories in every generation to "prove" that poverty can be overcome by anyone willing to work hard—in a nation whose economic system *requires* systemic poverty (un- and underemployment) as much as it requires consumers. If we think of domestic ideology as a network of social roles on the model of the family, in the national family African Americans have been assigned the role of domestic servants whose underpaid work keeps the household functioning—a metaphorical configuration with a very literal history in the United States.[40] Thus, regardless of how clean the homes or how industrious the families of the Lower Ninth Ward, the "blackness" and poverty of the population intersect in our nation's ideological network to suggest laziness, dirtiness, and incapability. Even as domesticity's (il)logic is acting to justify the exclusion of the Lower Ninth's former residents from the "new" New Orleans, it is serving the same purpose it served in Victorian England: to facilitate the exercise and consolidation of power by political and business leaders in New Orleans, who stand to benefit from having a wealthier, whiter population in the post-Katrina city.

Their policies are creating a New Orleans that will be very different, demographically, from the New Orleans we lost. According to sociologist Gary Perry, as of late summer 2007, "an astounding 73 percent" of the pre-Katrina African American population had not returned.[41] Some of those who could have done so chose not to return to a place where "we're not wanted" or where the post-Katrina opportunities and services are so thin.[42] Many are eager to return. But too many post-Katrina policies are likely to ensure—by design or in practice—that the city's racial majority will not be black again.[43] For example, in the months immediately following the storm, the Lower Ninth was singled out by Mayor Ray Nagin and others in city planning discussions as a neighborhood that should not be rebuilt. Undeniably, there were defensible arguments to be made for turning the land, which was originally a cypress swamp, into a public green space. An important point was that rebuilding in a highly flood-prone area would put residents in danger of future flooding; however, the same was true of Gentilly, a less black, middle-class area, and Lakeview, a wealthy white community, and their rights to rebuild were not fundamentally challenged.[44] Then, only one month after Lower Ninth residents were first permitted to set foot back in their neighborhood, the city began making plans to demolish several of the buildings in the area. Again, real public safety concerns justified the proposed step—the buildings scheduled for immediate demolition were considered structurally unsound and likely to fall in ways that could potentially kill or injure people and damage adjacent structures. But a number of factors indicated that the city was insensitive to or uninterested in issues of equity raised by its decision: for example, the city initially deemed homeowners to have been put on notice of the demolition by the red stickers it placed on the doomed houses, *despite* the fact that large numbers of the residents remained in postevacuation exile all over the country. Further, as residents began to challenge the plan, they discovered that houses that had not suffered structural damage—completely recoverable buildings—were among those that had been selected for bulldozing. These problems suggested to some that the urgency of the demolition plans was intended to demoralize those who are committed to returning and rebuilding the Lower Ninth.[45]

Consider these events in light of what is happening with the city's four largest public housing complexes, St. Bernard, C. J. Peete, Lafitte, and B. W. Cooper. Despite desperate need for affordable housing and over the protests of current and former residents, the city has razed three out of four public housing complexes, and the razing the fourth was under way as of January 2009 to make room for "mixed-income" housing. The 4,500 units will be replaced with fewer units, the majority of which will be rented at unsubsidized prices that will exclude the people who once lived there.[46] The majority of the existing units were not damaged by the flooding; nevertheless, in the initial months after the floods receded, housing authorities refused to allow residents back into livable units, instead spending $500,000 to board up, fence off, and demolish public housing.[47] Because redevelopment projects involving New Orleans's public housing complexes were already occurring or on the table before the storm, policymakers argue that Katrina only sped up the process. But others have argued that to take the hurricane-related evacuation as an opportunity to displace thousands of people permanently from their homes, all at once, is not just insensitive, but further evidence that the vision of New Orleans going forward does not include former residents who were poor and black.[48] The rhetoric used by several different politicians to discuss this issue invokes the conceptions of race, class, and gender that domestic ideology underwrites. Signally, U.S. Representative Richard H. Baker, from Baton Rouge, was quoted as having said that "[w]e finally cleaned up public housing in New Orleans. We couldn't do it, but God did," suggesting that empty or even flood-polluted apartments were "cleaner" than they had been when occupied by low-income African American families. (His remark also carries the dubiously religious implication that Katrina was an act of God which, like the Flood that only Noah's ark-full of creatures survived, was intended to rid the area of an immoral people.) New Orleans City Council President Oliver Thomas raised the stereotype of blacks as lazy (and thus not among the "deserving poor") when he proclaimed that "only those who want to work are wanted back in New Orleans' projects. The city doesn't need 'soap opera watchers.'"[49] Peggy Wilson, then a mayoral candidate, referred repeatedly to "welfare queens" in her campaign, which, since the beginning of the last quarter of the twentieth century, has been a derogatory label for women, especially African American women, on public assistance.[50] Thomas's and Wilson's comments connect gender and race in the demonization of black women who are able to be stay-at-home mothers with the assistance of the government; the same ideology perversely commends white and middle-class mothers for not working *and* condemns black, working-class mothers for leaving their children at home in order to go to work at financially necessary jobs.[51]

Putting the Lower Ninth Ward and the public housing complexes side by side, we can see that, whether lower-income African Americans live in flood-prone areas or on higher ground, whether they own or rent, they are struggling to prevent the city from evicting them from their former homes—and from the city entirely. The terrifying fact is that the logic of domestic ideology lends support to their exclusion in either case. The apparent inescapability of domestic ideology's racist applications is another type of violence that, like the forms of physical violence discussed earlier in this chapter, contributes to the circulation of gothic homelessness in African American culture. This is certainly true of those trapped by, or helplessly watching, its operations in post-Katrina New Orleans city planning. The ultimate irony revealed by comparing the fates of the Lower Ninth and public housing residents is perhaps also the ultimate example of gothic homelessness. The very people whose belonging in the "national family" was thrown into question when they were prohibited at gunpoint from leaving New Orleans are the same ones—predominantly African American and poor—who are now being prevented from returning to their haunted houses, the only homes they have known. Their very palpable absence will continue to haunt New Orleans, just as the horrors of Katrina's aftermath will feed the social terror circulating in African American culture for the foreseeable future.

NOTES

1. R. David Paulison quoted in Martin Kasindorf, "Nation Taking a New Look at Homelessness, Solutions," *USA Today*, October 12, 2005, http://www.usatoday.com/news/nation/2005–10–11-homeless-cover_x.htm. Michael Kunzelman, "5th Circuit Upholds Razing of N.O. Public Housing," WWLTV.com, January 27, 2009, http://www.wwltv.com/topstories/stories/wwl012709cbrazing.b321afe.html.

2. Gary Rivlin, "Casinos Booming in Katrina's Wake as Cash Pours In," *New York Times*, July 16, 2007, http://www.nytimes.com/2007/07/16/business/16casinos.html?_r=1&oref=slogin. For 2009 statistics, see Brookings Institution, *The New Orleans Index: Tracking the Recovery of New Orleans and the Metro Area*, https://gnocdc.s3.amazonaws.com/NOLAIndex/NOLAIndex.pdf.

3. "Editorial: Haunted by Disaster a Year after Katrina," *The Oregonian*, August 29, 2006, sunrise edition; Peter Whoriskey, "Silence after the Storm: Life Has Yet to Return to Much of a City Haunted by Katrina," *Washington Post*, August 27, 2006, final edition; Gwen Filosa, "Lower 9 Residents Differ on Desire to Return," *New Orleans Times-Picayune*, August 24, 2006, http://www.nola.com/newslogs/tpupdates/index.ssf?/mtlogs/nola_tpupdates/archives/2006_08_24.html#175830.

4. John Nichols, "Barbara Bush: It's Good Enough for the Poor," *The Nation*, September 6, 2005, http://www.thenation.com/blogs/thebeat?bid=1&pid=20080.

5. For an audio recording of the interview quoted herein, which aired on the radio show *Marketplace*, see "Houston, We May Have a Problem," *Marketplace*, September 5, 2005, http://marketplace.publicradio.org/display/web/2005/09/05/houston_we_may_have_a_problem/html. For a written account, see "Barbara Bush Calls Evacuees Better Off," *New York Times*, September 7, 2005, http://www.nytimes.com/2005/09/07/national/nationalspecial/07barbara.html?ex=1188619200&en=11cc1dace8f56ff8&ei=5070.

6. Nancy Armstrong, *Desire and the Domestic Novel* (New York: Oxford University Press, 1987), 82.

7. Anne McClintock, *Imperial Leather: Race, Gender, and Sexuality in the Colonial Contest* (New York: Routledge, 1995), chap. 10.

8. Evie Shockley, "Buried Alive: Gothic Homelessness, Black Women's Sexuality, and (Living) Death in Ann Petry's *The Street*," *African American Review* 40, no. 3 (2006): 439–460.

9. While the phrase "Katrina diaspora" was used commonly enough in reference to the dispersed New Orleanians in the months after the storm to make it a convenient shorthand for me here, under a precise definition of the term, the Katrina survivors who were then scattered across the United States would not necessarily constitute a diaspora—if only because their exile from New Orleans has not yet been of a long enough duration. See Kim D. Butler, "Defining Diaspora, Redefining a Discourse," *Diaspora: A Journal of Transnational Studies* 10, no. 2 (2001): 192.

10. Hortense Spillers, "Mama's Baby, Papa's Maybe: An American Grammar Book," in *Black, White, and in Color: Essays on American Literature and Culture* (Chicago: University of Chicago Press, 2003), 218.

11. Gary A. Donaldson, "A Window on Slave Culture: Dances at Congo Square in New Orleans, 1800–1862," *Journal of Negro History* 69, no. 2 (1984): 63–64.

12. Andrew Buncombe, "'Racist' Police Blocked Bridge and Forced Evacuees Back at Gunpoint," *Independent*, September 11, 2005, http://www.independent.co.uk/world/americas/racist-police-blocked-bridge-and-forced-evacuees-back-at-gunpoint-506371.html.

13. "Act II," *When the Levees Broke: A Requiem in Four Acts*, DVD, directed by Spike Lee, (HBO Home Video, 2006).

14. Buncombe, "'Racist' Police Blocked Bridge" ("Witnesses said the officers fired their guns above the heads of the terrified people to drive them back and 'protect' their own suburbs"); "Act II," *When the Levees Broke* (Vanita Gupta, assistant counsel for the NAACP Legal Defense Fund, discusses the fact and significance of the Gretna police officers calling the group of New Orleanians "thugs").

15. Associated Press, "Calling Katrina Survivors 'Refugees' Stirs Debate," MSNBC, September 7, 2005, http://www.msnbc.msn.com/id/9232071/; Mike Pesca, "Reporter's Notebook: Are Katrina's Victims 'Refugees' or 'Evacuees?'" NPR.org, September 5, 2005, http://www.npr.org/templates/story/story.php?storyId=4833613.

16. "Act III," *When the Levees Broke.*

17. Pesca, "Reporter's Notebook."

18. Associated Press, "Calling Katrina Survivors 'Refugees.'"

19. Pesca, "Reporter's Notebook."

20. Gregg Zoroya, "Return of U.S. War Dead Kept Solemn, Secret," *USA Today*, December 31, 2003, http://www.usatoday.com/news/nation/2003–12–31-casket-usat_x.htm.

21. Nicole R. Fleetwood, "Failing Narratives, Initiating Technologies: Hurricane Katrina and the Production of a Weather Media Event," *American Quarterly* 58, no. 3 (2006): 774.

22. Leon R. Litwack, "Hellhounds," in *Without Sanctuary: Lynching Photography in America*, ed. James Allen, 8–9 (Santa Fe: Twin Palms Publishers, 2000).

23. James Allen, ed., *Without Sanctuary: Lynching Photography in America* (Santa Fe: Twin Palms Publishers, 2000).

24. Fleetwood, "Failing Narratives, Initiating Technologies," 773–774.

25. While there are, of course, black people and other people of color in the military, and there were white people trapped in New Orleans during and after Hurricane Katrina, blacks do not constitute anything remotely approaching a majority of those in the military, nor did whites represent more than a minority of those stranded in New Orleans. The point, however, is not about majorities. The distinction between the two groups is a matter of both race and class—not in an economic sense, but rather in the sense of the military as a privileged class, especially in relation to blacks. Blacks soldiers may access a certain elevated status associated with the military, but the two— military and blacks—are distinct social categorizations, even if the membership of these two groups overlaps.

26. Baird Helgeson, "Disaster Tourism Begins to Thrive," *Tampa Tribune*, December 30, 2005, http://www.tampatrib.com/MGB9ZZ9oUHE.html.

27. For example, see http://www.neworleanskatrinatours.com.

28. Rolf Potts, "In New Orleans: The Allure of Disaster Tourism," Traveling Light: The Art of Independent Travel (blog), March 13, 2006, ttp://travel.news.yahoo.com/b/rolf_potts/rolf_potts2915;_ylt= AiU6o2Gp_KWuj6.

29. Helgeson, "Disaster Tourism."

30. Coco Fusco, *English Is Broken Here: Notes on Cultural Fusion in the Americas* (New York: New Press, 1995), 40–41.

31. Ibid., 43.

32. M. S. Gabriel, M.D., letter to the editor, *New York Times*, September 13, 1906.

33. See Fusco, *English Is Broken Here*, 41–43 and 50–58, for a dismayingly long list of parallels to the display of Ota Benga, occurring primarily in Europe, Australia, and the United States, and a fascinating discussion of Fusco's work with Guillermo Gómez-Peña in their performance piece *Two Undiscovered Amerindians Visit . . .* (preserved as a documentary video titled *The Couple in the Cage*) (Third World Newsreel, 1993), in which they provocatively restage this history of people of color as spectacle in art and natural history museums in cities on three continents.

34. Helgeson, "Disaster Tourism."

35. Filosa, "Lower 9 Residents Differ."

36. Shaila Dewan, "Patchwork City: Road to New Life after Katrina Is Closed to Many," *New York Times*, July 12, 2007, http://www.nytimes.com/2007/07/12/us/nationalspecial/12exile.html.

37. For example, Herbert Gettridge Sr. explains his unwillingness to leave the Ninth Ward as a result of his having built the house he lived in there (Filosa, "Lower 9 Residents Differ").

38. Guilbeaux quoted in Filosa, "Lower 9 Residents Differ."

39. For a Katrina-related version of this idea, see Charles Murray, "The Hallmark of the Underclass: The Poverty Katrina Underscored Is Primarily Moral, Not Material," *Wall Street Journal*, October 2, 2005.

40. A comment made by Louisiana State Representative Cedric Richmond is eloquent on the aptness of my metaphor in the local context. Rejecting the claim that plans to raze most of the city's public housing complexes are intended to relieve misery resulting from "the concentration of poverty in New Orleans," he noted, "It was always concentrated. Because you can't get people to make beds and clean hotels if you educate them well and they expect a decent pay" (quoted in Julia Cass and Peter Whoriskey, "New Orleans to Raze Public Housing," *Washington Post*, December 8, 2006, http://www.washingtonpost.com/wp-dyn/content/article/2006/12/07/AR2006120701482.html).

41. Gary Perry, "New Orleans Survivors: A People without a Home," *Freedom Socialist* 28, no. 4 (August–September 2007), http://www.socialism.com/fsarticles/vol28no4/28406new_orleans.html.

42. "Act IV," *When the Levees Broke* (Tonya Harris, resident of the Lower Ninth Ward, speaking about the desire of industry and business to gain possession of land in that area even before the hurricane); Suburban Emergency Management Project, "Three Katrina Evacuee Stories," *Biot Reports*, no. 306, December 13, 2005, http://www.semp.us/publications/biot_reader.php?BiotID=306 (see especially the testimony of Doreen Keeler, para. 11, and Patricia Thompson, para. 9).

43. Robert D. Bullard, "A 20-Point Plan to Destroy Black New Orleans," February 1, 2006, in A Katrina Reader: Readings by and for Anti-racist Educators and Organizers,

http://cwsworkshop.org/katrinareader/node/160; Bill Quigley, interview by Amy Goodman, "As Police Arrest Public Housing Activists in New Orleans, Federal Officials Try to Silence Leading Attorney for Low-Income Residents," *Democracy Now!*, January 31, 2007, http://www.democracynow.org/article.pl?sid=07/01/31/1543227.

44. Ceci Connolly, "9th Ward: History, Yes, but a Future?" *Washington Post*, October 3, 2005, http://www.washingtonpost.com/wp-dyn/content/article/2005/10/02/AR20051 00201320_pf.html.

45. Kari Lydersen, "Fight Continues over New Orleans's Lower Ninth Ward," *NewStandard*, February 21, 2006, http://newstandardnews.net/content/index.cfm/items/2841; Rick Brooks, "Katrina Survivors Face New Threat: City Demolition," *Wall Street Journal*, August 9, 2007, http://online.wsj.com/article/SB118662045674092462.html.

46. Cass and Whoriskey, "New Orleans to Raze Public Housing"; Associated Press, "Feds Approve Demolition of Four New Orleans Public Housing Complexes," NewsFlash: Upto-the-Minute AP News Reports, September 21, 2007, http://www.natchezdemocrat .com/news/2007/sep/22/feds-approve-demolition-four-new-orleans-public-ho.

47. Perry, "New Orleans Survivors."

48. Bill Quigley, "Why Is HUD Using Tens of Millions in Katrina Money to Bulldoze 4,534 Public Housing Apartments When It Costs Less to Repair and Open Them Up?" *CounterPunch*, December 29, 2006, http://www.counterpunch.org/quigley12292006 .html.

49. Baker and Thomas quoted in Gwen Filosa, "Public Housing Still Empty: As Residents Clamor to Return, Officials Weigh Fate of Complexes," *New Orleans Times-Picayune*, April 9, 2006, http://www.nola.com/frontpage/t-/index.ssf?/base/news-5/11445656492 75850.xml.

50. Wilson quoted in ibid.

51. For a thorough and illuminating analysis of this stereotype, see Wahneema Lubiano, "Black Ladies, Welfare Queens, and State Minstrels: Ideological War by Narrative Means," in *Race-ing Justice, En-gendering Power: Essays on Anita Hill, Clarence Thomas, and the Construction of Social Reality*, ed. Toni Morrison, 323–363 (New York: Pantheon Books, 1992).

PART THREE

"Starting Over" in Post-Katrina America

9

Rebroadcasting Katrina

Blame, Vulnerability, and Post-2005 Disaster Commentary

KEITH WAILOO

JEFFREY DOWD

"What is clear," writes sociologist Philip Kasinitz, "is that whatever national consensus eventually emerges on Katrina—what went wrong and who is to blame—it will have been largely forged in the media, and, perhaps *by* the media."[1] Across the board, commentators have identified the media (by which we mean print media, television, and online coverage) as a crucial force in shaping public understanding of Katrina. In this chapter, we argue that the media story of Katrina was forged not only in the initial coverage of the event, but that it has continued to evolve with subsequent disaster coverage—with each new catastrophe in the United States (from wildfires to floods to a bridge collapse), prompting new and ever-evolving Katrina references.

Assessing this post-2005 coverage, we examine the ways in which Katrina remains a touchstone for disaster reporting and commentary, a process that will likely continue for years to come. Moreover, the changing lessons embedded in this coverage and the limits of those lessons provide an important study of the storm's continuing imprint. By paying particular attention to how news stories and editorials invoke Katrina, the following pages illuminate the ways in which media make sense of subsequent disasters and Katrina as well. Media, we find, do not so much forge any national consensus on the events of 2005; rather, coverage defines and redefines the parameters of debate about Katrina's meaning. Through a robust, unfolding, and unpredictable process, media shape the broader discussion about the nature of disasters—their human-made features, their natural origins, their genesis in individual bad choices, their disparate impact, and the extent to which poor leadership or prior policy decisions create the bedrock for present calamities.

In recent media coverage of natural disasters in the Midwest and western United States, journalists and commentators have frequently invoked six explanatory frameworks to account for why some people are more vulnerable to

1. Acts of God, nature's fury	How has the media, since Katrina, used the events in the Gulf Coast in 2005 to frame subsequent coverage of disasters?
2. "Human nature" (selfishness, not thinking in the long term, individual or collective)	A review of 280 print media stories in 2007 and 2008 reveals Katrina's imprint on later disaster reporting.
3. The attributes and choices (good or bad) of the victims themselves	Although Katrina's lessons continue to be invoked by journalists and commentators reporting on those events, the lessons cited fall into widely disparate categories.
4. The heroism, incompetence, or actions of individual leaders	
5. Failures of infrastructure, and public policy	Any news story that reports on a fire, flood, or disaster by invoking Katrina tilts the meaning and significance of Katrina in particular directions.
6. Longstanding variations in structural vulnerabilities	

FIGURE 9.1. Explanatory frameworks in media coverage explaining disasters.

disasters than others: (1) characterizing disasters as acts of God or nature's fury, (2) attributing these catastrophes to weaknesses in human nature, (3) pointing to the victims' attributes and/or choices, (4) citing neglect by individual leaders, (5) blaming political choices for infrastructure failures, and (6) discussing structural vulnerabilities (see figure 9.1). Although journalists employ all of these explanatory frameworks in accounting for these events and there has been an admirable growth in the complexity of the coverage, we find that coverage and invocations of Katrina tend to overemphasize the first five while paying far less attention to the sixth, and we argue, most important, framework. Whatever the preferred cause, coverage often presents each framework as its own story, without regard for their complex interconnections, which are, in fact, the crux of what shapes vulnerabilities in disaster.

This critique should be read not merely as a blanket criticism of media disaster coverage but rather, more significantly, as a study of the power as well as the limitations of mass media in explaining vulnerability to a broader public. Certainly, there are different kinds of media stories of disasters—some doing a better job than others—and not all coverage can, or should, focus on the larger historical, social, or economic roots of vulnerability. After all, no newspaper story can be expected to match the breadth of extensive academic study. Thus, in this chapter, we are not primarily concerned with what the media leaves out but with what media coverage does contain and how it frames larger social issues and understandings of vulnerability, what we call "looking upstream" of the event itself and its key actors to past decisions and public policy.

We examined newspaper coverage of three post-Katrina disasters, using LexisNexis to search for all articles on these later occurrences that mentioned Katrina. The three events—the 2007 Southern California wildfires, the August 2007 I-35W bridge collapse in Minneapolis, and the 2008 Midwest floods—yielded ninety-nine, one hundred, and eighty-one articles, respectively. Our analysis focused particular attention on how the lessons of Katrina were portrayed in each context. We find that, with its singling out of particular blameworthy individuals, the media tends to overindividualize large-scale social and institutional problems. But our study of Katrina and post-Katrina disaster coverage also argues that because Katrina has multiple uses as it continues to linger in the public mind, it provides an opportunity for more extensive discussion of structural issues. The commentary surrounding the I-35W bridge collapse provided a particularly strong—even if flawed—model of how disaster coverage, using the example of Katrina, might develop in years ahead. For it is in the coverage of the bridge collapse that we see glimpses of critique targeting not merely individuals—be they victims or politicians—but rather policy decisions, infrastructure weaknesses, and other such structural causes of disasters.

As sociologists Kathleen Tierney and colleagues note, the media often present the public with a distorted and sensationalized view of disasters. Persistent "disaster myths" emerge, as was seen both before as well as during Katrina.[2] One myth, for example, insists that catastrophes create public panic and mass social disorder. This is rarely the case, however, and media reports frequently exaggerate the extent of social turmoil after calamities. In addition, scholars have criticized the media for perpetuating racial stereotypes during disaster coverage—a phenomenon that became particularly evident during Katrina. Scholars argue that the media present such distortions for two key reasons. First, during a disaster, journalists are "pressured . . . to fabricate news on the spot for public consumption . . . condens[ing] complex social processes into dramatic soundbites."[3] And as anthropologists Arthur and Joan Kleinman note, "In their attempt to produce images of suffering for public consumption, the media reduced complex stories to 'a core cultural image of victimization'";[4] more specifically, as Adeline Masquelier comments, these images frequently tilt in one direction—emphasizing "the failure, inadequacy, and irresponsibility of the poor."[5] In addition to pressure on journalists to produce material for easy public consumption, Tierney and her coauthors also cite "reporting conventions that lead media organizations, particularly the electronic media, to focus on dramatic, unusual, and exceptional behavior, which can lead audiences to believe such behavior is common and typical."[6]

Much has been written about media sensationalism and the pressure of rapid, unreflective coverage that makes for the reproduction of easy stereotypes.

During Katrina, some criticized the (perhaps inevitable) inclination toward sensational coverage adorned with premature and unsubstantiated depictions of social disorder (many with their implicit and sometimes explicit frameworks of black pathology).[7] On the other hand, Katrina coverage was also praised for drawing attention to suffering and for holding political leaders accountable. In the eyes of some critics, a press that many derided as sycophantic and frivolous redeemed itself in 2005. This study moves beyond the (important) assessment of sensationalism in disaster coverage to look at how a wider range of reporting conventions frame disaster understanding.[8]

Not only is Katrina now commonly employed to help define and explain disasters, but it is continually reinterpreted with each new tragedy—bringing different features of the Katrina event back into public discussion. By following these subsequent events, we examine how media coverage sets the stage for framing new events by employing Katrina in multiple ways to frame debate about public issues—from the role of government, responsibility for death, taxes, the character of those victimized, to the nature of vulnerability. Mass media can help to present disasters as political issues, or they can present calamities as unfortunate, random events (as, for example, apolitical acts of nature). Each event we examine—wildfires, floods, and so on—provides a framing opportunity. Some, like the California wildfires, provoked a retelling of Katrina by focusing on the violation of the social contract and the failure of government to respond, to help people, to issue warnings, and to coordinate disaster responses. Yet other events, like the Minneapolis bridge collapse, focused on Katrina as a lesson about misplaced priorities and a call to shift public policies and spending priorities of government. The politicization of Katrina (itself a highly political event) has continued, therefore, in post-Katrina disaster coverage.

Part I. Wildfires and Floods: "Natural" Disasters and Individual Choices

Katrina coverage undermined the facile dichotomy between natural disasters and social calamities, and between the event itself and its social causes and effects. Yet, drawing lines between the "natural" and the "social" persists as a vexing theme in media coverage of subsequent misfortunes. As one commentary surrounding the bridge failure in Minneapolis notes, "A bridge collapse is far different from a natural disaster. Nobody expects politicians to prevent a tornado or an earthquake. But the government built the bridges, owns the bridges and maintains the bridges, so everyone expects them to keep bridges from collapsing."[9] Academics have argued that this type of dichotomous thinking is flawed because it misses how natural and unnatural forces always combine to shape the nature and effects of calamities.

Before Katrina, media coverage was often quick to invoke the act of God or nature's fury story line—often sidestepping issues of human blame and responsibility. This process of naturalizing disasters and storms in the 1970s, 1980s, and 1990s masked issues of political responsibility. Consider, for instance, these lines from an editorial published in the days after Hurricane Bonnie swept through Hampton Roads, Virginia, in 1998: "When storms inflict damage that overwhelms any state's reasonable efforts to protect and succor its own, federal relief is due. And time and time again, Americans voluntarily have helped those hammered by the only forces a secular age describes as acts of God. . . . [But] Bonnie's damage did not rise to the level of national calamity. Although federal aid would have been welcome, it wasn't necessary. FEMA [the Federal Emergency Management Agency] made the right call."[10] Although the editorial acknowledges the contradictions between thinking of hurricanes as "acts of God" in "a secular age," it nonetheless suggests that the storm itself (its "natural" features) ought to determine the level of federal response. But in the years since Katrina, this "act of God" coverage has changed—and below we examine how recent disaster reporting has been accompanied by discourses of blame.

Blaming the Victims: The Uses of Katrina in the Hurricane's Aftermath

The discourse of blame and the individualization of calamites has been a prominent aspect of disaster coverage in the years after Katrina, and often Katrina is used as a point of comparison to further this blame. This could be seen clearly in the wake of the 2007 California wildfires, where some commentators focused on the propensity of people (as in New Orleans) to inhabit vulnerable terrain.[11] One commentator saw obvious Katrina parallels: "But one thing that the wildfires share with Katrina is that both natural disasters were made worse by the propensity of people to build homes in high-risk areas."[12] This commentator seemed to suggest that the floods and fires themselves were not the problem; the proximity of people to levees in low-lying areas and people building homes in fire-prone regions were instead the key problems. Continuing with the comparison between the fires and Katrina, this observer noted, "Katrina's economic impact was magnified by development along the vulnerable Gulf Coast. Similarly, the wildfires have been particularly brutal in newly developed communities in fire-prone scrublands and dry pine forests."[13] Such commentaries exemplify how in recent years, some in the media have used Katrina as a touchstone for asking why people end up in these vulnerable situations; in the process of exploring these questions of vulnerability, such commentaries construct a broader story line about what we call "collective bad decisions" that place victims in nature's path.

Some journalists and commentators used the motif of collective bad decisions, portraying the California wildfires as proof of a "propensity" or human inclination to make ill-advised choices, to build in dangerous locations.

As another article noted, "One of Hollywood's prominent actresses [Jamie Lee Curtis] said no one should be surprised the fires are ravaging Southern California. 'We live in a drought, we build houses too close, and then we're shocked when this happens? This is not an act of God. This is an act of man.'"[14] It then follows that if bad choices on the part of victims cause disasters, victims deserve little sympathy.

Some wildfire stories went beyond themes about individual decisions and looked to larger social and climate patterns. For example, urban theorist and author Mike Davis, who has long studied the complex forces that shaped development of Los Angeles, was quoted in one news report as saying: "The move into the hills is for homes that are more affordable, but they are also more vulnerable. An inventory by University of Wisconsin researchers found that about two-thirds of new building in Southern California over the past decade was on land susceptible to wildfires." Davis noted, "You . . . drive out the San Gorgonio Pass, where the winds blow over 50 mph over a hundred days a year and you have new houses standing next to 50-year-old chaparral. You might as well be building next to leaking gasoline cans."[15] With this powerful analogy, Davis also pointed toward the goal of building safe, affordable housing as an alternative plan. Coverage like this, though rare, moved away from blaming human flaws to examining the intersection of natural and unnatural causes.

Arguments that overemphasized the problems with building in nature's way often pushed aside other explanations for why people live in vulnerable areas. The nature's path framework assumes, incorrectly, that vulnerability is best understood as an intrinsic quality of a certain geographic area—or, in other words, it assumes that location determines vulnerability. But as Karen O'Neill's chapter demonstrates, Mike Davis's point is often ignored: decisions far upstream of the disaster explain its social effects. Unable, amid the pressures of wildfire coverage, to take this long view, media coverage often limits our understanding of how these disasters take place to human propensities—that is, people's desire to live in dangerous zones and their obliviousness to the consequences. This coverage touches on only a very small part of the story. By offering a framework rooted in individualized human action, some media stories steer readers away from considering how decisions made within the business or the political realm can create the conditions for so-called natural disasters and direct them instead toward easy truisms about human nature.

Human Interest Stories and the Rewriting of Katrina

Much of the individualizing tendencies perpetrated by coverage of both the 2007 fires and the floods across the Midwest in 2008 involved focusing on the acts of heroism and on stories of loss and tragedy. Often framed as human-interest stories focused on the experiences of disaster victims, these reports drew several comparisons with Katrina's victims, deploying the new disasters as opportunities to recast Katrina's victims as unheroic and as morally blameworthy actors.

In the collective portraits of fire and flood victims, some stories invoked Katrina to point to the attributes and choices of the victims. As one California wildfire story noted, "Officials are calling these some of the worst wildfires that San Diego County has seen in modern history. More than 500,000 people have been forced from their homes. But there is also a unique feel to this natural disaster, a distinctly California style, and it is not just the constant presence of Gov. Arnold Schwarzenegger on the TV screens. Meaning: California is dealing with it."[16]

Other articles echoed this image of a "can-do" spirit. Covering the midwestern floods, one author highlighted the unique qualities of those affected. "Fortunately, solid midwesterners, many of whom survived the record-breaking floods of 1993, seem to take even disaster in their stride. Neighbors have helped neighbors, and some cleanup has already begun in places where the floodwaters finally began to subside."[17] During the wildfires, when asked about how Californians were handling the level of displacement, "Staff Sgt. Zell Evans surveyed the scene" where National Guard members moved through the crowd without weapons. "'This is real different from Katrina,' said Evans, who spent 45 days in New Orleans after the 2005 hurricane. 'Here? There's no fear, no pushing, no fighting. Everybody is calm. It's just a completely different situation.'"[18]

In using the Katrina analogy, such reports indirectly suggested that the characteristics of Katrina's victims were somehow to blame; in contrast, the media portrayed these sufferers as a calm, fearless, and "completely different" people, taking calamity in stride—without fighting or pushing. This same article goes on to report that George Biagi, deputy press secretary to San Diego Mayor Jerry Sanders, "said no visions of New Orleans danced in his head. 'That was a whole region,' he said. 'With this, a lot of people can stay with friends. This is just a part of the city. And neighbors are helping each other out.'"[19] In a backhanded gesture, such reports characterized Katrina victims (most of whom were, in fact, calm and took displacement in stride) against these positive examples.

Such human-interest stories and tales of calm and solid heroism deploy Katrina as a point of comparison, and in doing so continually rewrite the story of what happened in New Orleans and the Gulf Coast in September 2005. Perhaps even without intending to do so, media coverage of subsequent disasters not only remembered but also re-created Katrina and its victims in the minds of American citizens. Disaster coverage often unconsciously assigned unique moral qualities to a set of disaster victims and implied by contrast that some victims are more heroic or less morally equipped than others to cope with the disaster's effects.

Individual Leaders under Fire

Of course, another individuating tendency in disaster coverage derives from the focus on the behavior and actions of political leaders tested by the crisis. In singling out "leadership" and the coordinated direction of people and resources as a crucial factor explaining low fatalities, media overstate the role of individual leaders. One editorial on the California fires recalled, "And Californians have something that Louisianans, in particular those in New Orleans, didn't have when they needed it most: leadership, in this case from Gov. Arnold Schwarzenegger and the San Diego mayor on down. That there have been just five fatalities in an inferno that has burned an area twice the size of New York City shows what can result from clear and coordinated leadership."[20]

After the wildfires, the press praised officials up and down the chain of command and (again) comparisons with Katrina became a staple feature of such coverage. Commenting on the numbers who had fled the fires, one reporter noted, "More than 10,000 refugees packed San Diego's Qualcomm Stadium, where local officials appeared to be running an efficient relief effort quite unlike the disaster that Hurricane Katrina survivors found in 2005 at the Louisiana Superdome in New Orleans."[21] In some ways, the Katrina story—with its dramatic failures to deliver emergency aid—set a low bar for leadership in subsequent disasters. Politicians, then, could evoke Katrina to claim improvement and to mask the other structural failures that contributed to the disaster. As one reporter noted, "Bush and Schwarzenegger gave each other credit for what they described as the prompt and effective response of state and federal agencies that had kept the number killed by the fires low, though the inferno has devastated 753 square miles and will end up causing more than $1 billion in damage."[22] But Katrina could also be invoked negatively. After the Midwest floods, the media found plenty of people who unhappily drew analogies between their situation and that of Katrina's victims. "The federal response is nonexistent," said Frank Bruce, fifty-nine, who was rescued from his home "at the last minute" by a fire department boat after he refused to board a FEMA boat that would not also take his two dogs. "I'm about to put a sign out saying 'Louisiana North.'"[23]

Such reports focus on the presence or absence of services and aid, but without any attention to why disparities in aid exist. "In their vivid reporting yesterday on the conditions at Qualcomm Stadium in San Diego," noted one editorial, "*Post* reporters William Booth and Sonya Geis didn't have to mention the horror that was the Superdome two years ago for readers to draw a comparison. The 7,500 evacuees at Qualcomm have cots and tents, plenty of water and a variety of foods, arts and crafts for children, crisis counseling, meditation, yoga, acupuncture, and AA meetings for adults. In New Orleans, 24,000 people seeking refuge at the Superdome were bereft of food, water and hope."[24] Focusing on the arrival of cots and vague proclamations about leadership and coordination, the media again personalized disaster coverage, but the details of the contrast (24,000 versus 7,500 refugees; the presence of cots versus the absence of any services, including electricity and clean water) were seldom examined deeply—that is with attention to the class, racial status, privileged status, and claims to services associated with citizenship in a first-world nation. Instead, quick characterizations of leadership, services, and people defined this post-Katrina coverage.

When individual politicians became the focus of disaster coverage in the years after Katrina, it was most often the superficial public relations features of their leadership—the performative aspects, the controlling of public perceptions, and the shaping of the political impact of the calamity—that were highlighted rather than disaster management per se. Thus, after the Minneapolis bridge collapse one newspaper article invoking Katrina remarked: "Unlike during the aftermath of Hurricane Katrina, when Bush was criticized for not visiting fast enough, the president quickly scheduled this trip to Minneapolis. He was expected to meet with victims' families later in the day. In the days after Hurricane Katrina battered the Gulf Coast in August 2005, President Bush was captured twice in photographs that have haunted him since: strumming a guitar in California and peering from a window of Air Force One as he made a low-flying pass over New Orleans on his way to Washington."[25]

Bush's leadership after the bridge collapse was presented as being in stark contrast to his public behavior following Katrina: "But on Saturday, the president will exhibit the faster, more direct response he has shown during national calamities since Katrina, personally touring the scene in Minneapolis where an interstate highway bridge collapsed."[26] In such accounts (and there were numerous articles echoing this theme), the public relations aspects of disaster leadership became elevated above all others. Moreover, Katrina was invoked as an event that provided a new yardstick for measuring the quality of leadership. Mayors, governors, and bureaucrats were judged according to this new leadership benchmark. Media commentators themselves became intimately familiar with this new, post-Katrina definition of leadership. Noted one source, "Since Katrina, Bush has also been alert to the public relations dimensions of disaster response, making an array of visits to the victims of wildfire, tornadoes, flooding and—in Minneapolis last year—bridge collapse."[27] In focusing on individual leaders, and in prioritizing merely the public relations aspects of leadership, much post-disaster coverage did not discuss (for example) how decisions leaders made before the event shaped its outcome. Administration officials themselves understood the new post-Katrina atmospherics. For instance, FEMA arranged a stage-managed press conference complete with fake reporters lobbing softball questions to FEMA officials in order to manage perceptions of their relief efforts during the California wildfires.[28]

Of course, such superficial discussions of individual leaders (their incompetence or their "leadership" gauged by their public relations moves) steer readers away from the historical patterns and structural realities that define vulnerability, as the chapters in this volume highlight. Though the media might focus on leadership in the wake of the calamity, few reporters delve into concrete political decisions made and the role that government philosophy plays in creating vulnerability. Instead, most stories may point vaguely to forces in the distant past (discrimination and racism in Katrina, for example) while ignoring entirely the role of distinct public policy in creating vulnerabilities and in maintaining the inequalities that shape the impact of disasters. Leadership matters, but President Bush alone was not responsible for bridges collapsing, wildfires erupting, levees breaking, or for flooding in the Midwest. Beyond criticizing individual leaders, we need to ask how flood, housing, fire, relief operations, and ecological management policy are shaped by particular policies created by particular administrations—thus determining the larger social phenomena of who is vulnerable and why.

Part II. Looking Upstream for Answers: How the Minneapolis Bridge Collapse Reframed the Infrastructure Debate

The shocking collapse, during rush hour, of the I-35W Minneapolis bridge over the Mississippi River on August 1, 2007, again brought Katrina back into the news, this time with commentators stressing the human-made dimensions of these calamities. The bridge collapse, more than the wildfires and floods, prompted a more complex debate about the roots of disasters. The obvious infrastructure failure was seen as a public policy debacle in which a system, rather than any particular individual, drew scrutiny. In particular, media coverage focused on earlier decisions, with reporters suggesting that disasters are made worse and people are made more vulnerable because of poor disaster planning, underfunded infrastructure, and lax regulations. Certainly, there was a focus on individuals affected and the personalities of leaders, but news stories moved quickly to "upstream" issues—the political and policy decisions that laid the groundwork for the catastrophe. Yet, as we will show, even this coverage showed the limitations of how media understands the role of class and race in shaping vulnerability in such events.

The bridge collapse was not an isolated event but "'a slow, creeping cancer that's been taking over the country,' said Ralph Dusseau, of Rowan University in Glassboro, N.J. 'Until something like this happens you don't see the disease.' In the days following the Minnesota disaster, transportation experts invoked Katrina—wondering why the failures of Hurricane Katrina weren't enough to prompt comprehensive infrastructure repair."[29] Such reports sought, at first, to place blame on government officials, but (failing to find easy culprits) disaster coverage often pointed to a general social failure—a failure of collective responsibility. "'I thought the wakeup call would've been the blackout or Katrina,' said

Patrick Natale, executive director of the American Society of Civil Engineers. For such observers, the bridge collapse provoked frustration about the pace of systematic reform. 'I fear,' remarked Natale, 'this incident will be like those. Time will pass and we'll forget.'"[30]

Frustration aside, the bridge collapse in Minneapolis provoked—more than the fires and floods—an expanded discussion of long-term infrastructure maintenance. Editorials cited Katrina and subsequent disasters as proof of a large-scale, lingering, and ignored set of social problems that formed the basis for disasters and that required prompt attention. One editorial argued, "The nation's physical foundations seem to be crumbling beneath us. Last week, a 40-year-old interstate highway bridge collapsed in Minneapolis, plunging rush-hour traffic into the Mississippi River 60 feet below. Two weeks earlier, an 83-year-old steam pipe under the streets of Manhattan exploded in a volcano-like blast, showering asbestos-laden debris. And two years before that, substandard levees gave way in New Orleans, opening the way for the floodwaters of Hurricane Katrina."[31] In the aftermath of this event, the Katrina tragedy could become part of a litany of infrastructure problems our society has neglected.

Rather than personal attributes, like calmness, competence, or concern, media reports evaluated the political decisions of the nation's leaders and turned to the impersonal and somewhat unglamorous question of how priority-setting by the government in the past could cause such disasters. Here, one also begins to see the seeds of another line of media analysis—the argument that spending priorities are not accidental, that there is a political logic shaping how such funds are disbursed, and that disasters have a deep historical relationship to choices about investing in infrastructure.

An important theme in media coverage—especially evident in the post–bridge collapse discussions—was the focus on the damage caused by past policy decisions, whether those decisions related to waging war, reluctance to raise taxes, or the prevailing "something for nothing" ethos that dominated American politics. As one author alleged, "The Bush administration's top priority, of course, has been its unending war in Iraq, which now costs $10 billion a month and is expected to consume $1.5 trillion to $2 trillion before all American troops are brought home. Everything else—from infrastructure to food safety inspections to the federal cops on the street program—has been slashed to pay for the war and tax cuts for the rich."[32] For some commentators, the bridge collapse followed clearly in the wake of tax policy: "The American Society of Civil Engineers . . . [had] concluded in 2005 that it would cost $1.6-trillion over five years to upgrade the nation's infrastructure. But most of its recommendations for financing the upgrades, including an increase in the federal gas tax, have been ignored."[33] Another writer in Virginia echoed this argument: "The federal gas tax hasn't budged in 14 years. In Virginia, where the idea of raising a gas tax to fund transportation needs was shunned in favor of new funding schemes such as abusive-driver fees, the tax on regular gasoline hasn't changed in 20 years."[34] In this view, the "real responsibility" for the calamity rested with those who were not willing to pay for improvements "based on the belief that we should get something for nothing." Who were the main culprits? According to one editorial, "Citizens who sign no-tax pledges are literally appealing to the common denominator of a free ride."[35] Not surprisingly, such arguments took on dramatic policy significance in Minnesota where, early in 2008, the state legislature "after the deadly bridge collapse in Minneapolis last August, enacted a law . . . raising its gas tax by 5.5 cents per gallon."[36]

Considering all these factors, media and public framing carried direct policy impact. Noted one commentator, "it has taken five years and $7.4 million to get a controversial tax plan to pay for regional road improvements on the fall ballot, and, until this week, many people believed it would be a tough sell at the polls." The bridge collapse altered the dynamics suddenly and dramatically— leaving (he hoped) a lasting imprint on priority setting and on the policymaking process. "As was the case in the aftermath of Hurricane Katrina, voters this fall will once again be marking their ballots with images of destruction potentially caused by aged infrastructure vivid in their minds. Some experts say that may be enough to firm up support for a $16 billion tax package that will be essential to paying for a replacement of the state Route 520 Bridge and other highways in King, Pierce and Snohomish counties."[37] Invoking Katrina, the bridge collapse coverage repeatedly highlighted the flawed political priorities of government and stressed that lack of disaster preparedness was not simply a matter of uncaring or incompetent officials but instead was best explained by competing political interests, tax and spending priorities, and so on.

For some observers, the problem of neglected infrastructure was the very problem highlighted in the chapters by Roland Anglin and Karen O'Neill in this volume—the problem of federalism, or how the division of powers between states and the federal government could foster inaction, confusion, and abrogation of responsibilities. "The larger problem of crumbling roads, bridges and levees and crashing electrical grids can almost always be traced to a lack of investment," noted one author. "When budgets are tight, elected officials find it convenient to cut back on maintenance and leave some future administration to deal with the consequences. When Congress appropriates money for public works, the legislators typically prefer shiny new projects that will enhance their reputations, not mere maintenance on a bridge named after someone else." And when maintenance money is tight at the federal level, the states are asked the pick up the slack with unfortunate consequences. "The federal government has particularly lagged in paying for infrastructure projects, leaving state and local governments to assume the dominant role."[38] For some, then, the bridge collapse over the Mississippi exposed this large policymaking process—one in which systematic relationships rather than individual actors created erosion, decline, and planted the roots of disaster. As one commentator in California noted, the lessons of the I-35W bridge and of Katrina extended throughout the nation: "Often taken for granted, public facilities in Monterey County are being steadily eroded by a conspiracy of advancing age and the mounting heritage of neglect only partly stemmed by revenue-static local governments."[39]

The bridge collapse, more than the wildfires and floods, prompted a more complex debate about the roots of disasters. Although, as shown above, the bridge failure triggered a rich infrastructure debate, because of the proliferation of generic images of disaster victims, this event raised few questions about variations in structured vulnerability. Indeed, the stock nature of the images of victims of this rush-hour disaster—involving children on a school bus, middle-class car-owning commuters, and so on—presented a picture with which the so-called average American could identify. As one city resident recalled one year after the calamity, "Every time that I pass over a bridge or go underneath one, I am reminded of how lucky I am to still have my life. . . . I was on a section of the bridge that did not collapse, only to be five cars away from the edge that did."[40] These images and the kind of identification they invoked diluted some of the power of the many pointed critiques of infrastructure raised within media responses to the bridge collapse.

Varieties of Vulnerability: Affluence and Poverty

Each disaster provides different possibilities for understanding questions of race, class, and vulnerability. Within the context of the I-35W disaster, in which an array of commuters died or suffered, class and race did not exist as crucial determinants of who lived and who died. The bridge collapse (covered as a random tragedy) provided little opportunity to examine society's assumptions about the disparate impact of structural failure or about whose structures (levees, bridges, and buildings) should be maintained and whose can be allowed to deteriorate. Yet, despite the absence of obvious class and racial gradients in the story, the disaster did in fact raise important questions about how the media frames issues of vulnerability and collective responsibility regarding shared systems.

Coverage of the bridge collapse, like wildfire coverage, often sought to contrast those affected by explicitly referencing their difference from Katrina's victims. At times, for example, coverage during the California wildfires (the first major disaster after Katrina) stressed the organized behaviors of Southern California's affluent refugees. The individual faces of this calamity were starkly different from those in Katrina. As one observer noted, "In New Orleans most of the victims were poor blacks with no way to escape the floodwaters who crowded into the fetid Superdome and waited days for help. In San Diego, many of the area's 10,000 evacuees waiting out the crisis at Qualcomm Stadium drove there in nice cars. They appeared to be middle class and quickly began receiving food, blankets, board games, cots and pillows."[41] This story notes the contrast of poverty and relative affluence between the victims of the two disasters. One group drove themselves in "nice cars," the other crowded together waiting for public assistance. In the background of the story was a picture of disparate vulnerability (rooted in differential access to transportation), but such issues were not further examined. Shaped by Katrina coverage, the question turned to how government responded to such homegrown refugee situations.

In California's response to the wildfires, one editorial argued that the rapid response to emergencies was the product of longer-term planning—and, implicitly, not linked to the social status of victims: "Because of well-organized disaster preparedness planning at the state and regional levels and drills that are continually performed, California is considered the gold standard of emergency response. . . . After devastating fires in 2003, San Diego County invested in the automated reverse 911 system, which this week urged San Diego County residents to evacuate."[42] This investment in advance of the event (itself linked to the resources of the community), more than the individual qualities of victims, explained the orderly movement out of vulnerable zones, the calm expectation that help would soon arrive, and the relatively low number of casualties.

In some wildfire coverage, the relative wealth of individuals and communities was assumed to play a role—albeit an underanalyzed one—in the disparate outcomes. As one unusually incisive author commented during the wildfires, certainly the economic and property interests of developers, homeowners, and taxpayers figure importantly in the coverage. Indeed, the wildfires highlighted a long-standing debate among environmentalists, developers, and critics who knew that government policy heavily favored the developers: "Some of the areas hit hardest by this week's fires are near Lake Arrowhead in San Bernardino County. The area is thick with vacation homes, a sore spot for environmentalists who complain that federal taxpayers foot the bill for protecting houses near national forests." Thus did some critics (in the minority to be sure) point to choices made far upstream to develop these areas (ignoring the concerns of preservationists) as responsible for the disaster. And when disaster struck, the cost of such poor policies was ultimately paid by taxpayers who carried the heavy cost of protecting private property from fire, as some "50 to 95 percent of Forest Service firefighting costs went to protect private property."[43]

This article (particularly as a contrast with Katrina reporting) reveals the possibilities of disaster coverage for illuminating vulnerability and drawing a more complex picture of how the social structuring of poverty and affluence can both lay the groundwork for calamities. In general, Americans are more familiar with the recognition of poverty's link to vulnerability than they are with the connection between wealth and privilege and disaster-related vulnerability. The role of government in choosing sides and making policy (in California and in Louisiana), thus laying the groundwork for these events, is seldom explored systematically. Media coverage of disasters frequently assumes that wealth allows people to "fend for themselves" while poverty makes people dependent on government. While this formulation is not entirely false, as some coverage of the wildfires suggested, it oversimplifies the case—failing to recognize how the poor and nonpoor are both dependent on shared systems. In this portrait of vulnerability, which is all too rare in media coverage, vulnerability becomes not an attribute of an individual but a feature of a system that shields some from risk while leaving others in harm's way.

Conclusions

With each disaster, Katrina's lessons (and thus their imprint) in the national and local media are revised, a process that will surely continue because of the enduring symbolic power of the 2005 events along the Gulf Coast. From coverage of wildfires and floods to sewage breaks and bridge collapse, there has been an admirable growth in complexity of disaster coverage (partly because of Katrina, and mostly because Katrina has created an unavoidable template for reading all of these other events). However, Katrina has also provided journalists, columnists, and the media at large with many different frameworks for presenting the question of vulnerability. Despite the growth in complexity of coverage, we find that the American news media continues to tilt (perhaps inevitably) toward individuating these events—for disasters are, after all, disasters because of their impact on individuals.

Yet, in each catastrophe, the media have been capable of going beyond the traditional human interest stories—to investigate the roots of disasters. Although the urge has largely been to find individual culprits, nonetheless, in a fundamental way, Katrina has expanded the possibilities of media coverage of disasters. The reporting about Hurricane Katrina itself defied the normal script surrounding disasters, for Katrina reminded journalists that managing and preventing such tragedies required understanding the roots of calamities and the underpinnings of vulnerability, not only the uncontrollable forces of nature. Since August 2005, Katrina has not disappeared—these complex events have become a constant source for reflection whenever parallel events occur.

Despite this increasing sophistication, we find that the media discussion of vulnerability is still limited in important ways. The media—while increasingly able to explain the roots of disasters—have not advanced in their discussions of why certain people are more vulnerable to disasters than others. Intense attention to individual characteristics (of the victims and of those deemed to be "responsible" for the event) often crowd out and compete with these broader structural questions of vulnerability. In this context, Katrina's imprint on media coverage has yet to be felt.

Certainly, it is clear that Katrina shed light on poverty as one type of vulnerability. As David Shipler writes in his study of the working poor, "The poor have less control than the affluent over their private decisions, less insulation from the cold machinery of government, less agility to navigate around the pitfalls of a frenetic world driven by technology and competition. Their personal mistakes have larger consequences, and their personal achievements yield smaller returns."[44] Vulnerability (as the Minneapolis bridge collapse and the wildfires in Southern California make clear) is the result of social structures and decisions made upstream about those structures. Disaster coverage tends to lack this level of sociological analysis for obvious reasons—time, individuation, and the limits of space. Nevertheless, in a cumulative and largely implicit sense, as we have argued here, the media do in fact create an analytical framework for explaining disasters and vulnerability to readers. And unquestionably, in writing about disasters to come, journalists and commentators will invoke Katrina, thus continuing the process of remaking the event. We hope that, as that process unfolds, more attention is paid not only to the complexity of disasters' origins but to the complex disparities such events illuminate.

NOTES

1. Philip Kasinitz, "Katrina, the Media and the American Public Sphere," *Sociological Forum* 21, no. 1 (2006): 145.

2. Kathleen Tierney, Christine Bevc, and Erica Kuligowski, "Metaphors Matter: Disaster Myths, Media Frames, and Their Consequences in Hurricane Katrina," *Annals of the American Academy of Political and Social Science* 604, no. 57 (2006): 57–81.

3. Adeline Masquelier, "Why Katrina's Victims Aren't Refugees: Musings on a 'Dirty' Word," *American Anthropologist* 108, no. 4 (2006): 740.

4. Arthur Kleinman and Joan Kleinman, "Cultural Appropriations of Suffering in Our Times," in *Social Suffering*, ed. Arthur Kleinman, Veena Das, and Margaret Lock (Berkeley: University of California Press, 1997), 10. Quoted in Masquelier, "Why Katrina's Victims Aren't Refugees," 740.

5. Masquelier, "Why Katrina's Victims Aren't Refugees," 740. See also Merrill Morris, "A Moment of Clarity? The American Media and Hurricane Katrina," *Southern Quarterly* 43, no. 3 (2006): 42.

6. Tierney, Bevc, and Kuligowski, "Metaphors Matter," 61.

7. For example, see Earl Ofari Hutchinson, "Race, Lies and New Orleans," AlterNet, October 6, 2005, http://www.alternet.org/rights/26507.

8. Our focus on newspaper coverage is an attempt to get past the most sensationalized coverage, particularly that of the twenty-four-hour news channels, to what most would consider to be the most staid news medium—print journalism. In other words, a critique of media disaster coverage could certainly find ample material to disparage by citing Fox News, CNN, or even print sources like the *New York Post*, but here we look at the kind of media that tend to fall outside of the most egregious examples of problematic coverage—that is, we bypass the low-hanging fruit of media critiques.

9. Tom Webb, "Collapse Sends Shock Wave from Here to Washington," *St. Paul Pioneer Press*, August 6, 2007.

10. "Not a Disaster," *Richmond Times Dispatch* (Virginia), October 29, 1998.

11. Indeed, in the immediate aftermath of Katrina, many skeptics (including Homeland Security Director Michael Chertoff) pointed out that New Orleans is below sea level, insisting that the fundamental problem was not the hurricane itself but the very notion of building a city below sea level in a hurricane-prone region. To this, comedian Jon Stewart wryly retorted, "Well, there you have it, New Orleans is to blame for existing" (*The Daily Show with Jon Stewart*, video clip, September 7, 2005, http://www.thedailyshow.com/video/index.jhtml?videoId=125094&title=Headlines—Meet-the-F**kers).

12. "Different Natural Disaster, Same Risky Habits," *USA Today*, October 26, 2007, news section, 8A.

13. Ibid.

14. Corky Siemaszko and Nancy Dillon, "Millions Fleeing for Their Lives: Arnold Orders Mass Evacuation as Wildfires Rage from LA to Mex," *Daily News*, October 27, 2007.

15. Davis quoted in Karl Vick and Sonya Geis, "California Fires Continue to Rage; Evacuation May Be Largest, Officials Say," *Washington Post*, October 24, 2007, A01.

16. William Booth and Sonya Geis, "In the Great State of Serenity, Staying Cool amid the Flames," *Washington Post*, October 24, 2007, A01.

17. Editorial, "Our Hearts Are in the Heartland: Midwesterners, Fighting Floods, Are No Strangers to the Destructive Power of Nature," *Appeal-Democrat* (Marysville, California), June 19, 2008.

18. Booth and Geis, "In the Great State of Serenity."

19. Ibid.

20. "Not Another Katrina: Wildfire Response Shows Why California Is the Gold Standard," *Washington Post*, October 25, 2007, A24.

21. Siemaszko and Dillon, "Millions Fleeing for Their Lives."

22. Sonya Geis and William Branigin, "Wildfires Wane as Bush Visits California; Danger Remains, but Battle Is Being Won," *Washington Post*, October 26, 2007, sec. A.

23. Michael Abramowitz, "President Visits Inundated Eastern Iowa," *Washington Post*, June 20, 2008, sec. A.

24. "Not Another Katrina."

25. Mike Jaccarino and Carrie Melago, "Bush Hails Lifesavers, Vows Quick Fixup," *New York Daily News*, August 5, 2007, 4.

26. Mark Silva, "Bush Ratchets Up Response: Quick Minneapolis Visit Reflects Lessons Learned after Katrina," *Chicago Tribune*, August 4, 2007.

27. Abramowitz, "President Visits Inundated Eastern Iowa."

28. Al Kamen, "FEMA Meets the Press, Which Happens to Be . . . FEMA," *Washington Post*, October 26, 2007, A19; Spencer S. Hsu, "FEMA Official Apologizes for Staged Briefing with Fake Reporters," *Washington Post*, October 27, 2007, A03.

29. Katherine Reynolds Lewis, "Perils of Patchwork: U.S. Infrastructure Needs More than Money," *Post-Standard* (Syracuse, N.Y.), August 5, 2007, A4.

30. Michael Van Sickler, "Bridge Sounds Wakeup Call," *St. Petersburg Times*, August 5, 2007, B1.

31. "A Bridge Collapses," *New York Times*, August 5, 2007, editorial, 9.

32. "A Man-Made Disaster," *Chattanooga Times Free Press*, August 3, 2007, B6.

33. Van Sickler, "Bridge Sounds Wakeup Call."

34. "The Price of Ignoring Wake-Up Calls," *Roanoke Times*, August 6, 2007, B8.

35. Tom Holden, "Authority to Vote on Package Today," *Virginian-Pilot* (Norfolk, Va.), August 10, 2007, sec. local.

36. Damien Cave, "States Get In on the Calls for a Gas Tax Holiday," *New York Times*, May 6, 2008, sec. A, National Desk.

37. Chris McGann. "Collapse May Give Voters Incentive to Back Road Plan," *Seattle-Post Intelligencer*, August 3, 2007, A1.

38. "A Bridge Collapses."

39. Jim Johnson, "Safe Crossings: Local Bridges Safe, but Roads Need a Lot of Attention," *Monterey County Herald* (California), August 13, 2007.

40. Trisha Crichton, "I-35W Bridge Collapse: One-Year Anniversary, We Can't Forget," *Minneapolis Star Tribune*, August 2, 2008, 7A.

41. Daniel Wood and Candice Reed, "In Fire's Path, Lessons Learned," *Christian Science Monitor*, October 25, 2007, sec. USA.

42. "Not Another Katrina."

43. Vick and Geis, "California Fires Continue to Rage," A01.

44. David Shipler, *The Working Poor* (New York: Alfred A. Knopf, 2004), 7.

10

Protecting Our Assets

Private and Public Responses to Katrina

JOHN R. AIELLO

LYRA STEIN

Hurricane Katrina exposed a fundamental difference between private-sector and public-section preparedness and the divergent abilities within each realm to protect their assets and their people. For New Orleans residents in the last days of August 2005, the main concern for each and every one of the citizens was leaving the flooded city. Some left in their cars after the first storm warning, but many were left with no resources to evacuate the city and were, therefore, dependent on government services. The vice president of a large bank told us that "there was no problem in getting out of the city. . . . And then we got in the car. We dashed out of here." The easy confidence expressed by this executive was not shared by all business managers and owners.

In this chapter we contrast public- and private-sector ideas about protecting people and assets, and we present the Katrina experiences of a number of business owners who were able to marshal resources that were considerably greater than those available in the public sector. We focus primarily on their responses in interviews we conducted over the twelve months following this costliest hurricane in history.[1] Some companies had planned for a crisis, practiced disaster preparation, and built up resources in case of an emergency, but many small businesses—without access to the capital or the reserves on which others were able to draw—had no such ability to prepare. Although the scene of tens of thousands waiting at the Superdome for food, water, and transportation from the government is etched in the memory of our country, the complexity in private-sector responses bears deeper scrutiny.

The story of small business and the Small Business Administration (SBA)— both in the evacuation and in the recovery of New Orleans—is a particularly important one for understanding private-sector preparedness and the problem of leadership. In the face of the coming storm, many small businesses were just getting by from day-to-day sales. This reality has also shaped the recovery process. As one small-business owner noted, "If you've got the money, okay. I mean if you don't have the money, you can't get back in business. The banks won't loan you the money. SBA can't get to you. I mean the crisis, the magnitude of it is that if my place had burned down to the ground, I would be further along." For many of these business owners, government agencies like the SBA and the Federal Emergency Management Agency (FEMA) were just as crucial for the process of returning to normal as such agencies were for private citizens. Small businesses are the "economic engine" that drives the recovery effort.[2] With small-business recovery acting as the rousing energy in the economic recovery, the SBA is integral in this effort. However, as another business owner noted, "I have applied for a SBA disaster loan and have been turned down twice. . . . It's a catch-22, you see. They say that, well, with the things that are going on, and my financials, and showing that in the past eight months how bad things have been that I couldn't pay the loan back. And I'm saying, 'But, hello! Isn't that what a disaster loan is for? To get you through the times until you can get back up?'" Small businesses had to negotiate a complex bureaucracy. If a business was unsuccessful and rejected by the SBA and did not receive any money from insurance coverage, it could apply to FEMA for a disaster recovery loan. But, a business could only seek FEMA assistance if it was denied an SBA loan, and it took about three months to receive a response to the application. In addition, if one was denied an SBA loan, it took additional time for this denial to be processed by FEMA.[3]

Small-business owners expressed many of the types of frustrations with this system as did the private citizens struggling to recover. Those who were able to evacuate the city and had the resources to take action early had a much different experience than those who were not as fortunate: "I actually got a very nice loan. I got a $250,000 loan, secured by my worthless house. . . . The breach was on the 30th? I think my application was the 31st. And I stayed online, in fact I got online, got halfway through, it was three o'clock in the morning. I kept trying. Nobody could get in. I kept trying this. I said, 'Well, nobody's going to be up at three o'clock in the morning.' . . . They did the entire application at about five a.m. for me on the cell phone."

However, the failures of government that were all too familiar to Americans watching FEMA were also evident to small-business owners. The SBA was not equipped to deal with the magnitude of the situation. The local SBA was flooded out of its office. Therefore, beginning the recovery process was a monumental undertaking from the start for small, fragile businesses. For those who were vulnerable and needed the immediate capital to begin to revive their profit margin, assistance without delay was crucial. As one owner noted, "If we don't get help within the next couple of weeks, we will have to move out of Louisiana and start over elsewhere. . . . Our savings, now seriously depleted as we await an SBA loan, may last a few months at best. Our applications for loans and grants has been buried under red tape, and now we are forced to consider leaving the city in which we grew up and love."[4] Another owner commented that "the government's not sending you any money. You could apply for the SBA loans, but they can't even come close to responding to the situation. The banks are all devastated." Thus, once again, the lack of leadership and organization had a spiraling effect on the city. The beacon of hope for the future of fiscal recovery was itself ill-equipped to rejuvenate an economically devastated New Orleans. The SBA was greatly overburdened with applicants, and an outreach program was initiated to acquire more personnel just to make way through the backlog of applications.[5] Those businesses, waiting patiently, with the hope that the government would come through, were often let down once again.

From the perspective of business owners, where federal agencies failed, there were state programs that could support their vulnerable businesses—but these too proved to be problematic. The state of Louisiana allocated revenue for a "Bridge Loans Program" to help businesses get back on their feet. These loans were allotted specifically to facilitate the survival of operations while owners were awaiting approval from various financial assistance programs. These loans were interest-free for 180 days and ranged from $5,000 to $25,000 per small business. Although they were beneficial for small-business recovery and maintenance of operations, the short-term nature of the loans created other difficulties, as another businessperson explained:[6] "And then I . . . took the bridge loan from the state and then paid that back when I got the SBA loan and got another loan. Right now I've got 100,000 in loans, which I have to pay back in September, and that's really what I'm using as my working capital. So that'll just come out of my savings. But for the first part we were just living this nightmare of using my insurance money."

The overriding atmosphere in the city was that of being left in the dark with no direction and no confidence that conditions would turn around. There was no hope that businesses and individuals would be given the means to rebuild from the ground up, especially those who lacked the resources and depended on the government to facilitate the recovery. "They gave me three weeks of business interruption coverage. They allowed me three weeks. But the business interruption started September 1st. And I said, 'Well how in the hell can you start business interruption September 1st, when we were under a mandatory evacuation order until October 1st? Shouldn't we have coverage through September, plus three weeks of October?' Nope." Bills were due, but there was no income. One small business owner complained, "Overnight we lost 12 percent of our sales. . . . If we are not able to plug this hole, we won't be able to employ the same number of people."[7] Even the businesses that survived Katrina unscathed lost their clientele and were left on unstable ground—but some small businesses were more vulnerable than others.

Disparate Impacts by Race

For minority business owners who already had a difficult time maintaining their businesses, the recovery process was even more complex. Before Katrina, minorities made up 36 percent of Louisiana's population and owned 14 percent of the firms in the state, but minority businesses represented only 1.8 percent of total sales and 2.7 percent of the total payroll.[8] More than three-quarters of minority-owned businesses started with no borrowed capital. In addition to the lack of financial capital, they also lacked social capital, such as ties to the Rotary and familial resources, as well as education, experience, and market access.[9] The disparate possession of resources needed for recovery left those who were more susceptible to breakdown even more vulnerable.

The result of those disparate business vulnerabilities has been evident in the years since Katrina. Of the African American business owners interviewed two years after the storm, 78 percent indicated lower earnings than before Katrina, compared with 60 percent of Caucasian business owners. In addition, African American business owners indicated that they worried about their demand market more than either Caucasian or Latino business owners did. They had more difficulty in being afforded credit, with 40 percent stating that they had trouble, compared with 28 percent for Hispanics and 25 percent for Caucasians. In a survey of the disconnection of business telephone services, African American businesses had a 28 percent higher rate than Hispanic-owned businesses and nearly 110 percent higher than Caucasian-owned businesses.[10] Lastly, Orleans Parish, the area hardest hit by the storm, contained the greatest number of African American businesses pre-Katrina. Consequently, African American businesses may have been impacted to a greater extent than other groups.[11]

Many factors played a role in this discrepancy in business recovery. Studies show that businesses located in predominantly African American markets are likely to serve low-income customers.[12] Because the citizens of New Orleans who evacuated after the storm were minorities of low socioeconomic class, African American businesses lost the majority of their clientele. Most of these businesses were in the service industry and catered to tourists, whose presence in New Orleans immediately disappeared right after the storm. The shortage of minimum- to moderate-wage workers created additional hardships for the businesses in the tourism and entertainment industries. The lack of adequate staff certainly affects whether a business can survive. "So life after Katrina has cut down the locations. . . . I don't have as many employees, and secondly, I don't have the business. . . . If business doesn't return, then there's no long-term survivability. . . . It's very difficult and basically because we've been so tourist-oriented."

Minority business owners faced additional challenges in the recovery process. Most of them were too small for venture capitalists and too risky for banks. As such, they had to rely on government help. However, many of the government programs and rules designed to ameliorate the disadvantages faced by minority businesses were suspended or relaxed. About 1.5 percent of the $1.6 billion awarded by FEMA has gone to minority businesses, less than a third of the 5 percent normally required. The government also eased affirmative action rules for contractors.[13]

Woodrow J. Wilson, the principal owner and manager of Gulf South Animated Technologies, a minority-owned small business in New Orleans, presented his concerns before the Senate Committee on Small Business and Entrepreneurship. He stressed the importance of giving minority-owned businesses funds to hire city and urban workers, who do not have many specialized skills. Minority-owned businesses, he claimed, are the "heart and soul of places like New Orleans," and without the jobs they create, inner-city workers will still be "in a trap and dependent." Minorities have long been a major contributor to the music and hospitality industries and contribute substantially to the unique cultural climate of New Orleans. Without the directed assistance to small minority business owners, New Orleans may lose that which "makes it New Orleans."[14] Additionally, the creation of jobs in New Orleans could reduce the pre-Katrina poverty level. Wilson said, "If the recovery effort wants to use Louisiana businesses, I have safety products and medical supplies, tools and pharmaceuticals and many things that may be needed for the cleanup. We just hope some Louisiana companies will be able to [work] as contractors and subcontractors on the actual work."[15] Socrates Garrett, an African American owner of Garrett's Construction, was sure he would get work after Katrina. He registered on FEMA's Web site and called companies hoping to get work removing debris, but had not received any contracts. "These guys," he said, "haven't given me a single bite."[16]

One implication of the recovery process was this: the federal government's suspension of regulations regarding contracts and bidding hurt small and minority businesses. First, government eased affirmative action rules for contractors. Furthermore, although local businesses usually get first crack at the bid and nonbid contracts, the government found loopholes that allowed it to contract with larger companies in the wake of Katrina. The Stafford Act provides preferences to locally owned businesses in contracting following a disaster and recognizes that contracts awarded to small, disadvantaged, and local businesses stimulate the local economy.[17] Under various federal laws, small and minority-, veteran-, and women-owned businesses receive preference to compete for contracts. While the government claims that it complied with the Stafford Act, it has used a loophole in the federal regulations to dole out federal contracts. A company can be counted as a small business even if it was once small; as a result, the government can still legally comply with the act if a business was classified a small business at one time, regardless of its present size. The government gave out lucrative, no-bid contracts for recovery work to large corporations by relying on the SBA's definition of small businesses—which vary from industry to industry.[18] One small-business owner, appalled at the way the Stafford Act had been corrupted, commented, "It's unbelievable. And for Bush to be down here, constantly saying, 'We will make you whole. We will rebuild this great city,' it's lip service. . . . 18 months later, nothing's happened. The Stafford Act has got to be blown up. . . . The red tape . . ."

Larger enterprises were not as vulnerable to the rapid shifts in the economic and regulatory climate—indeed, many were in a position to provide their own forms of assistance. Not all businesses lost everything in the storm; some had contingency plans. One man, Alden McDonald Jr., who had vast networking and political connections, took the steps necessary to stay afloat: "Mr. McDonald, the [CEO] of the largest black-owned bank in New Orleans, is relying less on tangible assets to help revive the banks fortunes; his many connections to people in powerful positions."[19] He made an effort to speak with top players in the government and lobbyists alike, not only about opening his bank but to make loans to the business owners in need of capital so they too could start to rebuild.[20]

In the unstable post-Katrina climate, with time being a crucial factor in business survival, connections and social networking proved critical for recovery. One business owner in the entertainment industry was fortunate enough to have connections within the community that helped restore his power: "One of the major, I mean the major, obstacle to get opened was to get electrical power. . . . Now that was an extremely difficult task that I was fortunate in being able to overcome. . . . We've got a very close friend of the family . . . he was an electrician. I begged him to put me at the top of his list. . . . I was fortunate that my brother-in-law . . . had contacts in electrical supplies in Lafayette. . . . And so from the time we started, it took about a week, and that's how I got power. So I had power hooked up October 30, which was very quick considering the circumstances."

The business was able to recommence, and "it was amazing I was getting the crowds that I got considering that you couldn't even call up to see if I was open." When he opened, shortly after Katrina, the media alerted the people who had come back to the city. Many flocked there as a refuge from the trauma. It was one place where people could relax, have fun, and forget the stress of their lives for a while. Though there are some examples of success stories, most minority-owned and -operated businesses were at a disadvantage owing to lack of resources and government manipulation of laws intended to help this demographic.

Contrasting Business and Government Capabilities in Evacuation and Recovery

While it has become commonplace to speak of the public sector's failure in Katrina, it is instructive to bear in mind the fundamental differences in private- and public-sector goals, missions, and leadership capabilities. By "leadership," we mean to draw attention to several key issues: (1) the lines of authority and empowerment of first responders, (2) the ability to stage resources, and (3) the anticipation of communications difficulties.

The Coast Guard and National Guard stand out as particularly bright spots in government preparedness and leadership. Given that in general the government response to Katrina was slow and unreliable, it is important to highlight those segments of the public sector whose response to the crisis was organized and competent. The National Guard took the lead in search-and-rescue missions and facilitated the immediate response. One small-business owner testified, "The National Guard, the military units, they were pulled out way too soon. Now there's still some here, but there's operations going in and cleaning up, and they came in, but they were so much more efficient than what's being done right now." The Coast Guard was also lauded for its ability to aid in the immediate response: "Like the Coast Guard . . . businesses prepared for this disaster by learning the lessons of previous disasters and by configuring their disaster preparation and response capabilities accordingly. They prepositioned their assets and personnel out of harm's way so that they would be available to deploy as soon as conditions allowed. They brought in assets and personnel from other locations to assist. They anticipated the failure of conventional communications systems and took measures to overcome those failures. And perhaps most important, they empowered their front-line leaders with the authority to make quick decisions and to take decisive action."[21]

Though the Coast Guard and the private sector were prepared and able to take action directly, there is a fundamental difference between the two. While the first priorities of businesses were related to the specific interests of the businesses—their assets as well as their employees and customers—many businesses were able to take on additional responsibilities, as Gary Rivlin noted: "The Coast Guard's core mission is to protect the American people. The core mission of a business is to maintain its operations and its ability to provide useful goods and services to consumers. But by protecting their assets and personnel, and by taking steps to restore their operations so quickly in the storm zone, these companies were positioned to help others and to serve society as a whole."[22]

There are shining examples of well-resourced preparedness in the private sector. A large petroleum company in the area had, according to one of its executives, "a very proactive system in place. . . . [With] Katrina coming, we had the

Gulf of Mexico completely evacuated in advance of the storm." Even after the hurricane hit, the company had the resources and the organization to hit the ground running. "We did make arrangements and brought in aboveground storage tanks so that we had fuel there and diesel for our generator. . . . We brought in forty-three trailers, temporary trailers from different parts of the country and set up basically three office complexes on site."

And although the government has come under harsh criticism for its handling of the aftermath of the storm, Wal-Mart is being held up as a "model for logistical efficiency and nimble disaster planning," which allowed it to come to the aid of the city. Wal-Mart offered $20 million in cash donations, 1,500 trucks of free merchandise and food, and the assurance of a job for all of its displaced workers.[23] The merchandiser made sure that all of its employees had money and a place to go. How was a large organization able to come to the aid of the citizens of New Orleans while the government, whose function is to protect its people, failed? Wal-Mart was prepared, had planned early, and made sure that the communication lines were open. It started its preparation operations on August 23, when Katrina was just a tropical depression. As soon as the storm showed up on the radar, merchandise was dispatched to stores, teams were staged, generators were brought in, and other preparative and alleviative actions were taken. In addition, it empowered its leaders with the authority to act. The store's director of business continuity explained, "For Wal-Mart, as far as the company reacts as a whole, we had total company support from our CEO all the way down and had twice-daily conference calls during Hurricane Katrina with the CEO, his direct reports and their direct reports and everyone knew that they would function through the emergency operation and use the structure that was in place."[24] In the White House report on the government's handling of the storm, "The Federal Response to Hurricane Katrina: Lessons Learned," one of the points emphasized was to "build a system and approach that better aligns authority and responsibility—those who are responsible for a mission or task must have the authority to act."[25] Success in the private sector can be attributed in part to the authority of the local teams to order anything needed and take whatever steps necessary to respond rapidly.

Stability became an overarching concern in a city threatened by anarchy, and it was the police (not businesses) who were best positioned to address this level of disorder. Much of the police force, to whom many look in times of need, had fled the city. "The sad part about it in New Orleans is there is no visible leadership anywhere. . . . The police, they had no leadership. They had lost their precinct, it was under water. Seeing anybody from the mayor to the governor to the president not there in the first few days . . . left anarchy in the city."[26] The anarchy and the looting that ensued after the storm led many police officers to give up or, on occasion, to join in the looting themselves; 91 officers resigned and 228 were investigated for leaving their posts. They were fighting a losing battle to take back a city that was spiraling downward fast, amid chaos and looting. As well, morale was at an all-time low, given that 70 percent of the officers lost their homes themselves. When the police communications went down because of troubles with the cell phone tower, each officer was on his or her own. One stabilizing influence was Deputy Chief Warren Riley, who deployed missions from the Hyatt Hotel. "I was just focused on leadership, trying to lead," Riley said. "I had officers tell me, 'As long as we hear you on the radio, we know we're going to be all right'"[27] For Riley, communication—in the immediate wake of Katrina—was crucial.

Communication continued to be paramount in the recovery of New Orleans—not only for policing, but for businesses as well. One of the most vital issues in getting a business back on its feet is the ability to communicate. Businesses that were able to contact each other, their vendors, and others outside of the city were able to network and begin the road to recovery. In the days following Katrina, communications were down as cell phone towers were leveled and land lines demolished. About 3 million phone lines were downed during the storm, and one thousand cell phone towers had to be restored.[28] The public sector, once again, was not prepared for the lack of communication to and from the city and within the city. The U.S. Senate hearing on what the government could learn from the private sector's response to the hurricane discussed, for example, "the picture of Mayor Nagin in a hotel room, no communications ability, one staff member has a personal computer, and over that computer, they hooked into . . . six or seven phone lines, and that was it for the Mayor of New Orleans."[29] Worse still, "During the course of time, for about 3 or 4 days, there was absolutely no communication whatsoever [from the government]. There was no support from a standpoint of military or anything else downtown that we saw."[30] The only working systems that functioned in the area were ham radios. Hundreds of amateur radio operators were deployed to the devastated regions to help provide critical emergency operation support. Most important, they played a major role in the rescue effort, connecting Red Cross facilities across towns.[31]

In addition, the Internet was literally a lifesaver for many in New Orleans. Without the resources to publish its newspaper, the *Times-Picayune* combined efforts with NOLA.com to publish online. Not only was the Internet a means of keeping citizens informed about the happenings after the hurricane, it served to reunite families and help rescue workers find victims. Postings to the Web site came in from around the country, alerting rescue workers to the locations of friends and relatives who were trapped in their homes, which the National Guard then used in its search-and-rescue missions.[32] Many calls for help were communicated using text messaging, given that cellular service was erratic. "The only way that we could communicate was by text messaging. Our cell phones weren't working. They were completely obliterated. The infrastructure wasn't working, so we were text messaging," said one small-business owner. Those companies that were prepared, and had the resources, worked around the lack of cell phone service in the area. For example, an executive at a large bank in the region "went out and bought Houston area code, 713 area code, cell phones . . . hundreds of them" and was able to maintain communications with its employees.

Communications companies—some of them intense competitors—began to work together in the wake of Katrina, in the name of public programming and charity. In an attempt to increase communication throughout New Orleans in the first few days after the storm, an association of radio stations formed the United Radio Broadcasters of New Orleans. This unification, which began on September 1, 2005, and was led by WWL-AM, was unique in that it involved the teamwork for two competitor media companies, Clear Channel Communications and Entercom Communications. In a noble act of leadership, these two rivals came together to share space, equipment, personnel, and broadcast programming catering to public service, which among other benefits, consisted of finding lost friends and family. In all, about fifteen stations combined programming to broadcast to the city and surrounding areas.[33]

Not all leadership in the aftermath of Katrina lacked cohesiveness (for example, businesses marshaling resources and filling the gap in charity, in communication, in philanthropy, and in recovery efforts). Charity, big business, and large corporations made their philanthropic mark immediately after the storm. One of our interviewees said, "Really it's people in organizations [who] give money to people in other organizations. And it was without question the social trust and interaction with people in other organizations that came to our aid. It was that social network that I think played itself out all over the place. So in our case, it was foundations that had funded us."

It was groups like nonprofit organizations that were able to fund-raise with affiliates throughout the country and aid people and businesses alike. Within a city without visible leadership, those who had the assets and the resources stepped into a void to help the people of New Orleans recover. One nonprofit group hired teams of rescuers and through a national Web site that it launched was able to get the names and addresses of those who were left behind or needed help. It managed to save fifty people during the first week and brought the survivors together for religious services to give these people a sense of community at a time when spirits were languishing: "The first need that we addressed was a listening ear and knowing that somebody's there for them. The immediate second need was financial, and we immediately began distributing money, which we were raising. We launched a fund within about thirty-six hours, and our national affiliates over the country were helping us with generating money, and we were able to distribute hundreds of thousands of dollars within those first few months."

One such organization that was uniquely qualified to deal with the need for immediate disaster funds was the Idea Village. The Idea Village, formed in 1999, is an economic development organization whose goal is to create a linked network of resources to assist the development of entrepreneurs. It had been a driver of business innovation supporting the growth of local entrepreneurial ventures for years prior to Katrina. After Katrina, the Idea Village was in a position to assist small businesses that were not able to obtain adequate funding elsewhere. The company formed the "Re-Build New Orleans" project, which consisted of four teams of MBA students from Tulane. This project, described as a "Peace Corps" for entrepreneurs, was a tour-de-force for helping companies obtain expertise in recovery. The first course of action was to find out where the businesses, the owners, and the employees were located. Once businesses were located, the project provided immediate funds until the SBA and insurance money came through. It raised $700,000 in private money, received 550 different applications for funds, and had given out 120 grants by of the summer of 2006. The key goal of the Idea Village was to rebuild a business within nine months of Katrina, because after that amount of time there was not much chance of recovery.

These examples illustrate that leadership depends not simply on the moral or intellectual qualities of an organization or individuals. Instead, leadership also relies on communications, the availability of resources, and the lines of authority that allow those resources to be deployed. Any one of these facets of leadership by itself is not sufficient. Rather, the combination of these factors determines effectiveness. Moreover, what becomes evident in this analysis is the existence of a gradient of leadership, not only from the private to the public sector but across each of these sectors.

Individual Efforts in Recovery

Alongside the overarching focus on government and business responses to the Katrina catastrophe must be placed the recognition that much of the leadership exercised in the midst of the disaster came from private individuals who found themselves on the front lines of evacuation and recovery efforts. Citizens were not merely passive victims waiting for others to lead, but in fact they were assuming leadership roles in the heat of the chaos. In the aftermath of Hurricane Katrina, the citizens of New Orleans were viewed as a population in need of the help of the government to be rescued from the devastation of the storm. Little attention was focused on the people of New Orleans as assets to the recovery process. FEMA began "preparations that ranged from logistical supply deployment to a mortuary team with refrigerated trucks."[34] However, the agency ended up failing the city's citizens. Many were forced to stay in the overcrowded Superdome and New Orleans Convention Center, with little food and water, awaiting buses to be taken out the city. Media outlets revealed the image of empty school buses waiting, sitting in water in part because Mayor Nagin wanted Greyhound buses.[35] Though the city only had enough buses to evacuate 10 percent of those needing assistance, even these limited resources were not utilized. Had the city been prepared, these vehicles could have evacuated many of those who did not have the resources, or were physically unable, to leave the city. The real heroes were the organizations and citizens of New Orleans, even if their response remained woefully insufficient with regard to a crisis of this magnitude.

From the wide-reaching efforts of organizations to ensure the safety of their employees—their most important assets—to the laudable efforts of private citizens who contributed to the recovery process, it was the citizens of New Orleans who demonstrated leadership. An owner of a bed-and-breakfast recalled:

> My husband and son searched for our employees. They literally went shelter by shelter for our valued employees. We have had people with us since we started, for twenty-one years. These people are part of our family. We were able to find twenty of them. . . . Ten only had the clothes on their back left. . . . We brought in hot meals, paychecks, and gasoline. I'm trying to care for two housekeepers and a maintenance guy, who were literally washed away by Katrina, and one housekeeper spent three or four days on a roof, had to be lifted off by helicopter. I feel responsible for these people.[36]

The focus of many organizations was on their employees. They realized the importance of treating their patrons as assets and made enormous strides to ensure that their employees and customers were safe and protected. Starwood Hotels started lining up buses after the levees failed on the Monday after Katrina hit. When the company heard that the levees had breached, it contracted buses from a private agency and was able to get its employees and guests out of the city. Starwood knew it had to evacuate instead of moving guests to the Superdome or the Convention Center, where no help would be found.[37]

Citizens became the real leaders in a New Orleans left in disorder—rescuing people and animals from life-threatening situations, mobilizing volunteers, clearing refuse, and so on. Where the government failed amid poor leadership and ineffective communication, a large network of rescue and emergency workers, along with volunteers, worked together to bring New Orleans back.

In an amazing feat led by Laura Maloney, the executive director of the Louisiana Society for Prevention of Cruelty to Animals (LA/SPCA), a private nonprofit organization that provides animal control for New Orleans, fifteen thousand animals in the city were saved through the efforts of animal groups and citizen volunteers who rose to the occasion. Maloney and her team's work began in late August, after Hurricane Katrina hit. After setting up at the Lamar-Dixon

Expo Center in Gonzales, Louisiana, Maloney's group began rescuing animals on the interstate, where buses were picking up stranded evacuees. As animals were not allowed on buses, the city was overwhelmed by the many stranded pets, some whom were chained to gates and had no chance of survival, if not for the heroic efforts of this organization. Maloney and her staff found animals on rooftops, animals trying to stay afloat in the floodwater, and those that were about to die of starvation. Maloney explained that she was able to continue through the agonizing moments by "staying focused in the mission, the greater good and focusing on what you can do instead of what you can't do."[38] She worked for more than a month without any days off, as she was haunted by the heartbreaking and unforgettable calls from owners looking for their beloved pets. "I felt guilty sleeping even a few hours, but I knew I can't continue without just a little. Images of animals in water, scared, and suffering play over and over again in my head." Maloney's remarkable and impressive dedication to rescuing animals earned her the City Business 2005 "Woman of the Year" award.[39]

Another example of leadership amid a chaotic New Orleans is that of Becky Zaheri, a stay-at-home mother, who mobilized more than ten thousand local, national, and international volunteers to bag and remove a quarter million tons of debris from the streets of New Orleans.[40] Volunteers came out of the woodwork to help with the grueling job of removing the refuse that covered the city. It was because of the initiative of its citizens that New Orleans would once again be the unique city it once was. Becky Zaheri said, "I drove home and saw all this litter and debris everywhere and it seemed like nothing was being done about it. . . . I was born and raised here and I wanted to see it cleaned up. I wanted it to be a place we'd feel good about."[41] Two years after the hurricane, Zaheri was concentrating on anti-litter awareness in neighborhood schools and businesses.

The main lessons learned from Katrina, for many businesses as well as for volunteers, have been the importance of taking disaster response into their own hands in case a catastrophe of this magnitude should occur again. Many businesses realized that success was based on the resources at their disposal. Preparing for such an event could mean anything from a small-business owner who "didn't take a thing other than my [computer] backup tape. I carried it in my pocket" to a large organization that had "planned for a long time in New Orleans because of the situation there with being below sea level and everything else. We all have our game plans at the beginning of the season, which is June 1, we have all our preparedness in place, and what happens is as soon as a storm is named, we start tracking it from that point."[42]

Just as there is a diversity in leadership capabilities, there is also (not surprisingly) a diversity in how businesses have recovered; this reflects a mismatch between resources and the needs of specific businesses. From the large companies that had disaster plans, which were rehearsed months beforehand, to the small companies, which only had to board up windows or remember their backup drives, businesses took proactive and widely divergent steps in preparing for the storm and responding in the aftermath. As one small-business owner noted, "I copied all the files from our server onto my laptop . . . all of the files with me. . . . My designer took backup files from the computer and took it with her to Cincinnati." New Orleans will be a stronger city given that the businesses that rebounded are the ones that had the ability to make it back or to stay open.

Some organizations were not so fortunate. For various reasons, many small businesses had to close their doors. These were usually ones that did not have the working capital to deal with recovery right after the storm or that relied on tourists to keep their heads above water. The owners of an automotive services business in New Orleans had to close their shop, which had been in the family for three generations, because business was so bad. They had to lay off all but two employees and decided that leaving the shop would likely give them something from their twenty-three-year investment, rather than continuing to lose money.[43] Another business, an electronics manufacturer, was forced to close because its insurance company refused to pay adequately for the damage to the structure and the loss of contents inside. "They have destroyed my business. I place more blame on the insurance company than the storm. They've destroyed my belief in mom and pop companies."[44]

One small bed-and-breakfast did all it could to revive its business and to acquire the funds to tide it over until tourists returned to the city. It did everything right: it had flood insurance, business insurance, and wind/storm insurance, but it could not bring in enough capital from these sources. The business insurance paid the owner nothing, the flood insurance paid enough to fix the air conditioner, and the wind/storm insurance had not paid anything as of December 2005. In addition to damage that made it impossible for the business to function, many patrons requested that their deposits be returned to them. After being turned down twice for an SBA loan, the owner did not know where to look for help. "How about being sixty-one years old and starting over with nothing—zero and I mean truly zero. It looks great, but nobody's going to pay what this place is mortgaged for in this town at this time. So that's it. I mean I'm talking everything. They've got my furniture. They've got everything. I have nothing. I virtually have nothing. If it all goes; you know, if they decide to really do a number on me, I just go get a shopping cart and [start] living under the interstate." Fortunately, through a network of innkeepers, who took up a collection over the Internet, the owner was able to receive some extra money to help with repairs and (it is hoped) drum up business.

Hurricane Katrina created a situation that divided the citizens of New Orleans into those who had the resources to evacuate and those who did not and had to rely on the government and other organizations to endure. The levees broke, the city was flooded, and the citizens were the casualties. Those fortunate enough to possess the resources to leave the city and the ability to rebuild were sharply contrasted with those left in the city after the flooding. Many of the organizations local to New Orleans, large and small, had the assets not only to help themselves, but also to help those who were suffering because of government ineptitude. Those who were not as well-situated (relative to key lines of authority, the communications system, the deployment of resources) were left in a state of lassitude and were barely able to meet their basic needs.

Comparing Public- versus Private-Sector Responses

For many people, the story of Katrina is the void of leadership—the mayhem and looting that ensued in a city that was left with little structure or direction. Through the darkness of downed power lines and waist-high floodwater, individuals and organizations came together to help where the public sector failed. These people and groups realized that the people of New Orleans were its greatest assets, and they set out to rejuvenate the city. They took up donations to save the unique character of New Orleans through rescuing those businesses that did not have the resources of their own to survive.

Many lessons learned from the events that occurred after Katrina can illuminate our understanding of preparedness, leadership, and the protection of assets. The public sector can learn a great deal from the response of much of the private sector, and vice versa. From the preparation to the response after the flood, there were numerous examples in the private sector of being geared up for this disaster. Many companies had preparedness plans that were not just written but were practiced, and as a result they were equipped to deal with evacuating and protecting their employees and assets. When the highest level of government failed to come to the aid of New Orleans, the state and local levels failed under that leaky umbrella. Help could only be found from those who were proactive and had a plan in place. The government learned a very hard lesson: that in the future it needs a means to evacuate those who do not have the resources to leave on their own. Considerations should also include providing a place for citizens to stay and provisions for food and water, if they are unable to get everyone out of the city. On the individual level, government should facilitate the education of its citizens in the preparations that can be made to plan how to leave the city and to procure a place to stay in a worse-case scenario.

Many organizations demonstrated that preparation was vital to surviving Katrina. "After Katrina left the city devastated, we were the first hotels downtown with power, trucked-in water, air conditioning and were the first hotels to open back up with restaurants. While some of the other hotels may have closed and evacuated their employees for weeks, we were able to accomplish these things because we had a plan, we had leadership, we had coordinated teamwork and because we communicated."[45]

In addition, many organizations and individuals found that an alternative means of communication was of the utmost importance. Simply backing up a computer or grabbing a disk on the way out was sufficient for some small businesses to survive. Many of the companies are now backing their work onto the Internet in case they are not able to return to the city for any reason. Just as the *Times Picayune* learned, the Internet was the saving grace of many people and organizations. Some businesses that were able to get online soon after Katrina actually experienced an *increase* in sales. "It was approximately mid-November [that I opened], and I did it solely because I felt that we would have good Internet orders and good customers for Christmas." Many had a crash course in how to use text messaging on their cell phones when cell reception was erratic. One company installed a 1–800 number so the dispersed employees would be able to call a central location.

While much of the public sector was mired in bureaucracy and could not communicate, it would be a mistake to ignore the diversity of effectiveness in both the public and the private sectors. As the case of the Coast Guard demonstrates, there is nothing intrinsic about the public sector or the private sector that makes one efficient and another inefficient in the face of such calamities. Although the disaster was widespread and devastated public resources, those with the assets were better equipped to weather the storm and recover from Katrina. Shell Oil was just one of those organizations that provided the resources to help bring the city back. Its support included the key sponsorship of the New Orleans's Jazz Fest even before the residents had returned to their beloved city. "Shell has taken a number of steps to actively assist in the area's recovery. In addition to returning its 1,000 strong employee base to One Shell Square early last year [2006], the company has also provided financial and volunteer support to a number of initiatives in South Louisiana since the 2005 hurricanes."[46]

These organizations buffered the inefficient response from the public sector. Though these efforts of businesses and individual citizens have aided in the city's recovery with their significant resources, their responses have been inadequate to help those who continue to be most vulnerable with regards the scale of this disaster. These vulnerable individuals will need more comprehensive private- *and* public-sector leadership to benefit from the recovery of the city and to weather the next storm.

NOTES

1. This research was supported in part by a Small Grant for Exploratory Research to the first author (and M. Doerful and I. Marsic) from the National Science Foundation. Interviews were conducted by the first author and M. Doerful. All quotations from business owners and others in this chapter are from these interviews, unless otherwise referenced. Interviewees gave permission for their statements to be included in

publications with the assurance that specific quotes would not be attributed to them as individuals.

2. U.S. Senate, *The Impact of Hurricane Katrina on Small Business: Hearing before the Committee on Small Business and Entrepreneurship*, 109th Cong., 1st sess, September 22, 2005, 46.

3. "FEMA Appeals," Katrina Legal Aid Resource Center, http://micdbgappeals.nixonpea body.com/shared%20Documents/Weil%20Gotshac%20Manges%20LLP%20FEMA% 20Asked%20Questions.pdf.

4. Quoted in ibid., 13.

5. U.S. Senate, *Strengthening Hurricane Recovery Efforts for Small Businesses: Hearing before the Committee on Small Business and Entrepreneurship*, 109th Cong., 1st sess., November 8, 2005.

6. "Louisiana Launches Hurricane Bridge Loan Program," Louisiana Economic Development Department, October 17, 2005, http://www.lded.state.la.us/press-archive/ 2005/10/20051017-louisiana-launches-hurricane-bridge-loan-program.aspx.

7. Quoted in Ken Belson, "Across the Gulf Region, Getting a Handle on What Comes Next; The Storm Missed Him, but Got His Customers," *New York Times*, September 20, 2005, http://query.nytimes.com/gst/fullpage.html?res2DA1630F933A1575AC0A96 39C8B63.

8. *The Impact of Hurricane Katrina on Small Business*. Prior to Katrina, New Orleans had a population of almost half a million, of which 70 percent were African American, significantly higher than the state average of 33 percent. Home ownership for African Americans was only 46.5 percent, lower than the state average of 68 percent.

9. "Katrina Impacts Tenth of Black Workers," Blackmoney.com, http://www.blackpress online.com/blackmoney.html.

10. Ibid.

11. Michael Turner, Robin Varghese, and Patrick Walker, *Recovery, Renewal, and Resiliency: Gulf Coast Small Businesses Two Years Later*, a Gulf Coast Economic Renewal Series Report by the Political and Economic Research Council, August 2007, http://www .infopolicy.org/pdf/Gulf%20Coast.pdf.

12. "Katrina Impacts Tenth of Black Workers."

13. Associated Press, "Minority Firms Getting Few Katrina Contracts," October 4, 2005, http://www.msnbc.msn.com/id/9590752.

14. Wilson quoted in *The Impact of Hurricane Katrina on Small Business*, 50.

15. Wilson quoted in Jackie Larson, "Gulf Coast Entrepreneurs Face Reality," *Entrepreneur*, September 22, 2005, http://www.entrepreneur.com/entrepreneurextra/features/article 80076.html.

16. Garrett quoted in "Show Me the Money: Minority Owned Firms Lag on Contracts," *U.S. News and World Report*, October 9, 2005, http://www.usnews.com/usnews/news/ articles/051017/17spotlight.htm.

17. *Strengthening Hurricane Recovery Efforts for Small Businesses*.

18. Griff Witte and Renae Merle, "Defining Small," WashingtonPost.com, October 20, 2005, http://www.washingtonpost.com/wp-dyn/content/article/2005/10/19.

19. Gary Rivlin, "Looking for Influence in All the Right Places," *New York Times*, October 18, 2005, http://www.nytimes.com/2005/10/18/business/18riberty.html.

20. Ibid.

21. Ibid.

22. Ibid.

23. Michael Barbaro and Justin Gillis, "Wal-Mart at Forefront of Hurricane Relief," *Washington Post*, September 6, 2005, http://www.washingtonpost.com/wp-dyn/content/article/2005/09/05/AR2005090501598.html.

24. Jason F. Jackson, director of business continuity, global security division, Wal-Mart Stores, testifying at U.S. Senate, *Hurricane Katrina: What Can the Government Learn from the Private Sector's Response? Hearing before the Committee on Homeland Security and Governmental Affairs*, 109th Cong., 1st sess., November 16, 2005, 29.

25. *The Federal Response to Hurricane Katrina: Lessons Learned* (Washington, D.C.: White House, 2006), 79–80, http://www.nola.com/katrina/pdf/katrina-lessons-learned.pdf.

26. *Hurricane Katrina: What Can the Government Learn from the Private Sector's Response?*, 19.

27. Riley quoted in Michael Perlstein and Lee Trymaine, "The Good and the Bad," *Times Picayune*, December 18, 2005, http://www.nola.com/crime/tp/index.ssf?/crime/stories/good_bad.html.

28. Caron Carlson, "Phone Companies Report on Katrina Response," eWeek.com, September 22, 2005, http://www.eweek.com/article2/0,1895,1862321,00.asp.

29. *Hurricane Katrina: What Can the Government Learn from the Private Sector's Response?*, 20–21.

30. Ibid., 18.

31. Gary Krakow, "Ham Radio Operators to the Rescue after Katrina," MSNBC, September 6, 2005, http://www.msnbc.msn.com/id/9228945.

32. Mark Glaser, "NOLA.com Blogs and Forums Help Save Lives after Katrina," OJR: The Online Journalism Review, September 19, 2005, http://www.ojr.org/ojr/stories/050913glaser.

33. Ibid.

34. http://www.safetycentral.com/hukadiinguco.html.

35. "Ray Nagin: School Buses Not Good Enough," Newsmax.com, http://archive.newsmax.com/archives/ic/2005/9/8/114045.shtml.

36. Quoted in *The Impact of Hurricane Katrina on Small Business*, 66.

37. *Hurricane Katrina: What Can the Government Learn from the Private Sector's Response?*

38. Maloney quoted in Jamie Guillet, "Laura Maloney Named City Business Woman of the Year," *New Orleans CityBusiness*, January 21, 2006, http://findarticles.com/p/articles/mi_qn4200/is_20060121/ai_n16019620.

39. Ibid.

40. "Katrina Krewe," Tulane University, http://www.newcomb.tulane.edu/NAfindingaids/KatrinaKrewe.html.

41. Quoted in "Trash-Talking Locals Pitch In to Clean Up New Orleans," FoxNews.com, May 15, 2006, http://www.foxnews.com/story/0,2933,195414,00.html.

42. Quoted in *Hurricane Katrina: What Can the Government Learn from the Private Sector's Response?*, 17–18.

43. Marlys Harris, "Coping with Katrina," CNNMoney.com, July 8, 2007, http://money.cnn.com/galleries/2007/pf/0708/gallery.katrina_pellissier.moneymag.

44. Quoted in Kathy Chu, "Katrina Still Wallops Small Businesses," *USA Today*, March 13, 2007, http://www.usatoday.com/money/smallbusiness/2007–03–13-business-insure_N.htm.

45. Starwood Hotels regional vice president of operations, Kevin Regan, quoted in *Hurricane Katrina: What Can the Government Learn from the Private Sector's Response?*, 10.

46. "Shell Extends Jazz Fest Sponsorship through 2010," Shell: United States, http://www.shell.us/home/content/usa/aboutshell/media_center/news_and_press_releases/archive/2007/jazzfest_extension_042807.html.

11

The Labor Market Impact of Natural Disasters

WILLIAM M. RODGERS III

Hurricane Katrina reignited debates about social policy and the role of government, particularly with regard to addressing racial inequality.[1] Media accounts as well as subsequent research have shown that African Americans bore the brunt of the storm, the failing levees, and the slow responses of local, state, and federal governments.

Most economic studies on major natural disasters examine the impact of a specific disaster by estimating the dollar costs of the destruction. For example, William Nordhaus, in his 2006 study of the economics of hurricanes in the United States, estimates that Hurricane Katrina and Hurricane Isabel (which hit North Carolina and Virginia in 2003) generated $81 billion and more than $3.3 billion of damage, respectively.[2] Yet, such studies have also found a hidden benefit after disasters. Studies that estimate the number of jobs lost find that losses in retail and other sectors are offset by growth in construction.[3] The recovery's length depends on the severity of the disaster and the community's economic health at the time it occurred. Healthier communities are more resilient than those that are impoverished.

When they strike, natural disasters are neutral to class, race, and ethnicity, but owing to residential segregation by income (which is correlated with the age of a community's homes, its infrastructure, and the amount of impervious surfaces) as well as income and wealth differences (which capture savings and access to credit markets), the impact of and ability to respond to the disaster may be more difficult for lower-income families.

Disparate impacts by race and ethnicity occur because minorities are segregated into older communities and have lower income (wages, weeks, and hours worked) and wealth. Thus, if the disaster is strong enough to disrupt an area's economic activity, low-income families bear the brunt of the losses. Because minorities constitute a disproportionate share of low-income families, they will have fewer resources and less access to the resources needed to recover. Thus, a profound recovery disparity exists in the wake of disasters like Katrina, highlighting the way in which vulnerability and inequality persist throughout the recovery process.

This chapter describes the racial differences in employment—one of several effects associated with Hurricanes Katrina and Isabel. First, I summarize published pre- and post-Katrina employment data for Louisiana and Mississippi. One difference between the two states stands out. Mississippi's aggregate employment was not adversely affected compared with Louisiana's employment. Much of this difference is the result of the dramatic decline in economic activity in New Orleans. Looking only at state-level data, however, masks what happened at the local level, in such places like Gulfport, Mississippi. Employment in Gulfport also fell as result of Katrina, but the drop was not as large, and the subsequent pace of the recovery has been quicker than in New Orleans. Furthermore, Gulfport makes up a smaller share of the state's overall employment, so its impact on the state overall was muted. By contrast, New Orleans's disaster had a more expansive impact on the state. After Katrina, Louisiana's African American employment fell more sharply compared with the state's white employment decline. Specifically, African Americans in New Orleans were disproportionately employed in occupations that contracted. For this reason, the storm had a disparate racial impact. Unfortunately, this is as far as one can utilize published Bureau of Labor Statistics and Census Bureau data to tease out the racial differences in Katrina's employment impact. Because of this severe data limitation, when considering Hurricane Isabel, I shift to utilizing my personal experiences—as a resident of Williamsburg, Virginia; as a board member of the United Way of Greater Williamsburg; and as a professional researcher—to describe that storm's disparate racial impacts. I conclude by identifying the characteristics of communities that could face the next Isabel, or worse, the next Katrina.

My overarching goals are to generalize the conversation about the disparate racial employment impacts of natural disasters and to provide a quantitative framework for future studies that will more rigorously estimate the employment effects of natural disasters.

The Macroeconomic Labor Market Effects of Hurricane Katrina

Natural disasters are categorized as severe storms, flooding, earthquakes, and tornadoes.[4] This chapter focuses on events that have been designated as major disasters, with the understanding that they are large enough to disrupt economic activity and have observable effects in the government data that I analyze.[5] Since 1953, an average of thirty Major Disaster Area declarations are made annually. Severe storms, floods, and hurricanes are the most prevalent

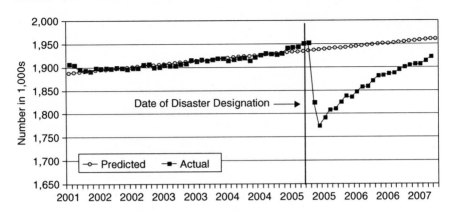

FIGURE 11.1. Louisiana Total Nonfarm Employment, November 2001–August 2007.

Source: Author's calculations from Bureau of Labor Statistics employment data. The trend line is fit using the data from November 2001 to August 2005.

declarations.[6] Here I examine labor market data before and after the major disaster designation for Hurricane Katrina. My analysis highlights how major job losses in New Orleans in all employment sectors other than construction dominate employment trends for Louisiana. Even several years later, employment losses had not been overcome in Louisiana. Comparing posthurricane job loss in Gulfport, Mississippi, versus New Orleans confirms that New Orleans has an outsize role in setting state employment trends.

Figure 11.1 shows a dramatic drop in total nonfarm employment for Louisiana.[7] In the two months directly following the designation of the Hurricane Katrina disaster, employment dropped from 1,950,000 to just below 1,800,000 workers. Employment has since risen at a faster rate than pre-storm trends, but overall employment remained below the September 2005 value as of August 2007.

Louisiana's sectoral response to Hurricane Katrina appears similar to responses found in studies of the effects of other natural disasters. While most major sectors contracted and have yet to return to their pre-storm levels, construction employment has accelerated and is above its predesignation trend line. Figure 11.2 indicates that Louisiana's construction employment dropped in the month immediately after the area received its disaster designation, but as of August 2007 more than twenty thousand new construction jobs had been added.

The manufacturing sector lost about 10,000 jobs right after the Katrina disaster, but a year and a half after the storm it had returned to its pre-storm value of about 155,000 jobs (figure 11.3). Because the pre-storm trends in manufacturing were trending lower, 2007 employment in this sector exceeded what would have been expected.

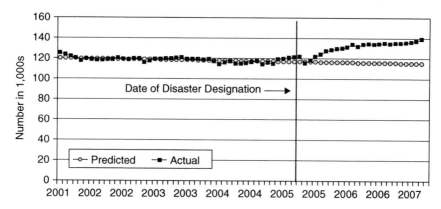

FIGURE II.2. Louisiana Construction Employment, November 2001–August 2007.

Source: Author's calculations from Bureau of Labor Statistics employment data. The trend line is fit using the data from November 2001 to August 2005.

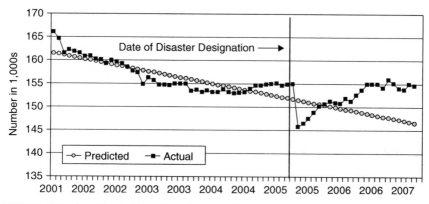

FIGURE II.3. Louisiana Manufacturing Employment, November 2001–September 2007.

Source: Author's calculations from Bureau of Labor Statistics employment data. The trend line is fit using the data from November 2001 to August 2005.

By contrast, the state's important leisure and hospitality sector, which shed about twenty-five thousand jobs in the two months after the storm, has since had steady growth, but total employment in this sector was still below pre-storm levels in August 2007 (figure II.4).

The data indicate that New Orleans residents bore the brunt of the storm. Prior to disaster designation, New Orleans's employment constituted between 31 and 32 percent of Louisiana's employment. In the two months following the storm this figure fell to 24 percent. During the remainder of 2005 and early 2006, the share increased, but leveled off at between 26 and 27 percent (figure II.5).

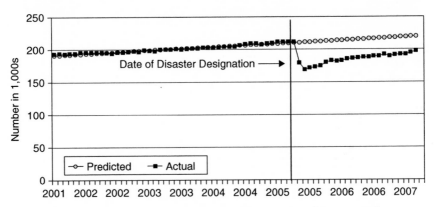

FIGURE II.4. Louisiana Leisure and Hospitality Employment, November 2001–August 2007.

Source: Author's calculations from Bureau of Labor Statistics employment data. The trend line is fit using the data from November 2001 to August 2005.

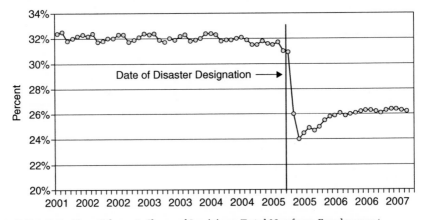

FIGURE II.5. New Orleans's Share of Louisiana Total Nonfarm Employment.

Source: Author's calculations from Bureau of Labor Statistics employment data. The trend line is fit using the data from November 2001 to August 2005.

In the two months following the designation, approximately 175,000 jobs were lost in New Orleans, dropping employment from just over 600,000 to 425,000 workers (figure II.6).

The vital tourism sectors (retail trade and leisure and hospitality) experienced significant job loss in New Orleans (figures II.7 and II.8). Retail trade lost almost thirty thousand jobs in the two months after designation. The good news is that two-thirds of these jobs returned by August 2007. In leisure and hospitality businesses, forty-five thousand jobs were lost in the initial two months after designation. Approximately one-half of these jobs had returned two years after the storm.

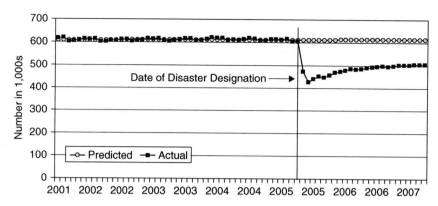

FIGURE 11.6. New Orleans Total Nonfarm Employment, November 2001–August 2007.

Source: Author's calculations from Bureau of Labor Statistics employment data. The trend line is fit using the data from November 2001 to August 2005.

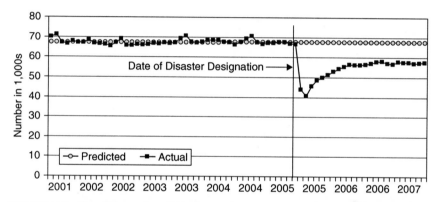

FIGURE 11.7. New Orleans Retail Trade Employment, November 2001–August 2007.

Source: Author's calculations from Bureau of Labor Statistics employment data. The trend line is fit using the data from November 2001 to August 2005.

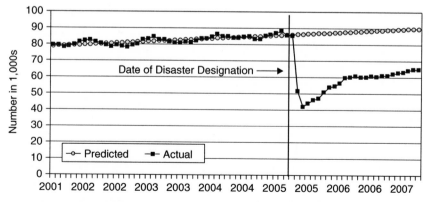

FIGURE 11.8. New Orleans Leisure and Hospitality Employment, November 2001–August 2007.

Source: Author's calculations from Bureau of Labor Statistics employment data. The trend line is fit using the data from November 2001 to August 2005.

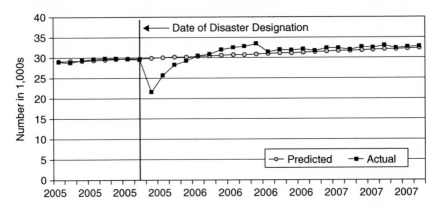

FIGURE II.9. New Orleans Construction Employment, January 2005–August 2007.

Source: Author's calculations from Bureau of Labor Statistics employment data. The trend line is fit using the data from November 2001 to August 2005.

In the month after the disaster designation, construction employment did fall, but it has rebounded (figure II.9). For several months it was above the area's pre-storm employment trend but subsequently returned to that rate. This leveling off, instead of a continuing acceleration, may explain why the other sectors have not returned to their pre-Katrina levels.

A major limitation of all these data, however, is that they do not indicate who obtained the new jobs: old or new residents. But it is well known that the city's population contracted. From July 2005 to July 2006, the New Orleans metropolitan area's population fell by 24 percent, from 1,312,400 to 991,902 people.[8] Data on racial differences in employment for New Orleans just prior to and after the designation are not available, either; therefore, I utilize two approaches that allow me to make some preliminary inferences. The first approach uses published annual data by race for Louisiana. The data have two major drawbacks: (1) Their annual nature prevents a direct comparison of employment levels before and after disaster declaration. (2) The figures are for the whole state rather than just the city of New Orleans. Nevertheless, the findings above seem to be solely driven by New Orleans. This means that the statewide annual series by race may contain some useful information about New Orleans.

In 2006, white and African American employment in Louisiana fell below their pre-Katrina trends. The drop has been larger for African Americans. Compared to one full year prior to the disaster designation, white employment fell by 2.6 percent, from 1,372,000 to 1,336,000 workers, while African American employment fell by 7.9 percent, from 533,000 to 491,000 workers (figures II.10 and II.11)

The second way to demonstrate disparate racial impacts is to show that at the time of the storm, African Americans were disproportionately employed in

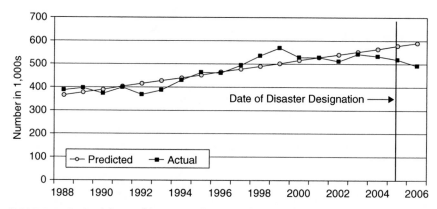

FIGURE 11.10. Louisiana African American Employment, 1988 to 2006.

Source: Author's calculations from Bureau of Labor Statistics employment data. The trend line is fit using the data from 1988 to 2006.

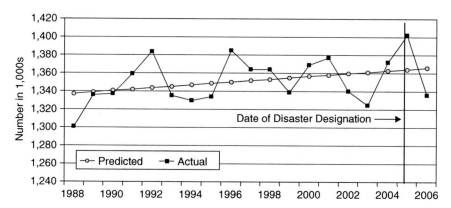

FIGURE 11.11. Louisiana White Employment, 1988 to 2006.

Source: Author's calculations from Bureau of Labor Statistics employment data. The trend line is fit using the data from 1988 to 2006.

low-wage occupations and that employment has shifted away from these jobs since then. The 2005 American Community Survey indicates that New Orleans's service, sales, office, and production occupations became a smaller share of New Orleans's employment in the four months after Katrina, while the share of jobs in management, professional, and related occupations increased. More specifically, the share of low-wage service occupations fell from 17.5 to 14.6 percent. The share of mid-wage sales and office occupations fell from 28.4 to 24.5 percent. The metropolitan area's share of high-wage management and professional occupations increased from 34.7 to 40.0 percent.

African Americans were disproportionately hurt by these shifts. In 2005, 25 percent of African American men were employed in service occupations, a

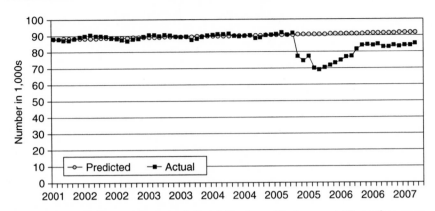

FIGURE 11.12. Gulfport, Mississippi, Total Nonfarm Employment, November 2001–August 2007.

Source: Author's calculations from Bureau of Labor Statistics employment data. The trend line is fit using the data from November 2001 to August 2005.

sector that had contracted, as compared to 11 percent of whites. Thirty-seven percent of white men were employed in management, professional, and related occupations, sectors that were expanding, versus 16 percent of African American men. More than one-quarter of African American women worked in service occupations in 2005. The comparable figure for white women was 14 percent. One-third of African American women were employed in management and professional occupations, as compared with 44 percent of white women.[9]

To explore whether New Orleans's employment patterns can be generalized to other Louisiana metropolitan areas, I examined Baton Rouge and Shreveport's employment data before and after the disaster designation (these data are not presented here). These areas suffered little, if any drop in employment, confirming that New Orleans is truly in a category of its own.[10]

In Mississippi, the impacts of the storm on employment were negligible at the state level. Employment fell in the month immediately after disaster designation, but returned to pre-storm trends and is now higher than its predesignation level. There are individual communities, however, where economic activity was impacted. For example, employment in Gulfport, which was hit heavily by the storm, fell.

Figure 11.12 shows that Gulfport employment had dropped five months after designation, leading to a loss of twenty thousand jobs. In 2006, more than half of these losses were recovered. As in New Orleans, employment in Gulfport has leveled off, so that in 2007, Gulfport was about five thousand jobs below pre-storm levels. Taken together, the data presented here show that New Orleans residents, and African American residents in particular, suffered greatly from job loss after Hurricane Katrina, and that these losses continue to affect Louisiana's economy in ways not experienced in other states.

The Microeconomic Labor Market Effects of Hurricane Isabel

For me, a natural disaster's ability to expose the intersection of race and class was a reality several years prior to Katrina. The second-most intense hurricane of the 2003 season, Hurricane Isabel, formed from a tropical wave on September 6, 2003, about six hundred miles west of the Cape Verde Islands.[11] As it neared the North Carolina coast and encountered stronger wind shear and cooler sea surface temperatures, Isabel weakened to a category 2 storm. It made landfall near Ocracoke Island, North Carolina, with estimated winds of 85 knots and then tracked northwestward before falling apart near Erie, Pennsylvania, on September 19. Rainfall amounts of more than six inches were reported in Maryland and Virginia. Isabel was responsible for thirty deaths, and insured damage was estimated at $1 billion.[12] The estimated overall damage was more than $3.3 billion.[13]

On September 18, 2003, Virginia's peninsula was formally designated a natural disaster area because of Hurricane Isabel.[14] At the time, I lived in Williamsburg, an area that was especially hard hit by the storm. For the nation, the storm and its aftermath garnered attention for a day or two; however, for Williamsburg residents, it served as a preview to Katrina. Williamsburg had neither faulty levees nor residents (largely low-income African Americans) stranded in William and Mary Hall (Williamsburg's version of the Super Dome and the Convention Center), but the area's location, economic structure, and patterns of racial inequality created the same risk factors as in New Orleans. Williamsburg is located on a peninsula bounded by the York and James Rivers. It has a high water table, and at the time of the storm, soils were saturated owing to previous rain. Several large, low-wage companies and sectors, including the College of William and Mary and tourism (Colonial Williamsburg, hotels, and restaurants) are the area's economic drivers. Large and persistent racial economic disparities characterize Williamsburg. In 2000, the typical African American family in Williamsburg had 80 percent of the typical white family income. In James City County, the county that surrounds Williamsburg, the typical African American family's income was 54 percent of the typical white family's.[15]

As a result of this income inequality, African Americans had significantly fewer economic resources to draw on in order to respond to the disaster. Although the outcomes were not as horrific as seen in New Orleans, Williamsburg's African American population was disproportionately affected by the storm. Destruction from the flooding and falling trees was debilitating to many residents, but especially to low-income African American residents. After the storm, most residents' electricity was out for one to two weeks. To minimize the likelihood of refrigerated foods spoiling, those with cars spent each morning trying to figure out where the daily shipment of ice would be delivered.

Assuming that they got there before the supply ran out, families were limited to two bags. Blue tarps sprang up on rooftops throughout the town to keep animals, rain, and insects out of homes damaged by fallen trees. Personal savings were drawn on to replace food, purchase generators, and pay for the removal of debris and subsequent repair of homes. Of course, the ability to respond in these ways depended on family resources and the labor market.

Getting Back to Normal

In Williamsburg, I saw numerous examples of how Hurricane Isabel generated disparate impacts according to race. Hourly paid workers were unable to return to work as fast as salaried workers. Many of the hourly jobs were in the retail and leisure sectors, including Williamsburg's vibrant tourism industry. Without electricity, these businesses could not operate. Tourists probably delayed vacations to Williamsburg until they felt that the area had returned to some semblance of normality. As a result, many hourly paid workers could not earn wages. On the other hand, salaried people like me continued to receive their paychecks. I, and others like me, could return to a modicum of normalcy more quickly than hourly workers.

Hourly workers tended to have low incomes and lacked savings, credit, and other resources, which made the labor market effects on income all the more drastic. In other words, the most vulnerable populations were the ones who lost jobs and income. A major difference that I observed between higher- and lower-income residents was how each group financed the replacement of food. Higher-income families utilized either savings or credit cards. Low-income families sought referrals from the United Way for local food pantries. This search for assistance was not a one-time event. At the end of the month, many of these families returned, seeking assistance with their utility bills. The storm may have started a downward spiral into poverty for some families who were living from paycheck to paycheck and had little, if any, insurance and savings. If not propelled into poverty, they were surely set back a few years in terms of accumulating wealth and savings for future expenditures such as financing their children's college education and their own retirements.

In an attempt to save perishables and maintain a semblance of normalcy, the middle- and upper-income response was to queue up at big box venders such as Home Depot to purchase a generator. Most low-income residents could not afford to buy a generator and then pay for the gas to operate it. To compound matters, African Americans, who were overrepresented among low-income residents, lived in older parts of the town where the power lines were above ground. Many of these neighborhoods also seemed to be at the end of the power grid. This added to the length of time it took for repairs.

Blue tarps and downed trees were present in virtually every neighborhood but had a prolonged and greater presence in low- and moderate-income communities. After the storm, the price of tree removal and general contracting services spiked upward for several months. As an economist, I marveled at how the market tried to solve the problem of tree removal. It took very little time for tree removal companies to descend on the area. Their outsider status was noticeable because the area codes of the phone numbers printed on the truck doors were neither Williamsburg's 804 area code nor Virginia and North Carolina area codes. Instead, I remember seeing Texas and Florida area codes. High-income families, those with savings and insurance, were the only ones who could afford to make immediate repairs. Likely, fewer African Americans had good quality homeowners' and storm insurance. For these residents, some companies offered cut-rate prices; however, those who used one of these services ran the risk of incurring further damage, because in this case the offered price was a "good" signal or predictor of the company's experience and insurance.

The Compounded Effects of Labor Market Impact

Why did African Americans bear the brunt of Hurricane Isabel? A primary reason, compounded by poverty, was the larger share of African Americans who worked as hourly wage workers. This made African Americans most vulnerable in Williamsburg, just as in the case of New Orleans. As summarized earlier, there are stark differences in income by race in the Williamsburg area. The median household income of African Americans in James City County was 54 percent that of whites. In Williamsburg, the comparable ratio was 80 percent. This figure is slightly deceiving because, on the one hand it obscures Williamsburg's several predominately white lower-income neighborhoods and on the other hand includes college students, who are predominately white.

The portrait of income inequality in Williamsburg further illustrates the community's "two realities." In James City County, 56 percent of African American families had incomes below $50,000, while only 29 percent of whites had family incomes below $50,000. In Williamsburg, the figures were even higher. Eighty-seven percent of Williamsburg's African American families had incomes below $50,000, as compared with 35 percent of Williamsburg white families. Poverty estimates for the area's children also provide an indication of why the storm had disparate racial impacts. The poverty rate of James City County's African American population was 23 percent, compared with 4 percent for whites. In Williamsburg, almost 50 percent of African Americans were in poverty, while only 19 percent of whites were below the poverty line.[16]

Were the adverse effects of Isabel long lasting? Published Bureau of Labor Statistics data indicate not; however, these data cannot be disaggregated by race. Overall employment in James City County and Williamsburg dropped in the month right after the region was designated a disaster area, but began to increase in the next few months. In James City County, it took only five months for employment to return to its November 2001–September 2003 growth trend. It took only two months for employment in Williamsburg to return to its pre-storm monthly trend.[17]

What Does the Future Hold?

Some scientists argue that the frequency and severity of natural disasters will increase as a result of climate change.[18] To minimize the general economic and social disruption and the disparate racial impacts, it is important first to identify the characteristics that placed Williamsburg and New Orleans at greater risk. Below are several significant economic characteristics:

- Low income and high poverty rates
- Low savings rates
- Poor access to insurance and credit markets
- Aging public infrastructures
- Unprepared and underfunded disaster preparedness programs
- Local and state budgets facing structural deficits
- Low public support for investing in community infrastructures
- Persistent racial and ethnic income inequality

Nordhaus identifies geographic areas in the United States with major concentrations of "at risk" economic activity and capital. They are the Miami coast, New Orleans, Houston, and Tampa. Lower-lying areas are at greater risk from storm surges and global warming.[19] Future work will integrate the economic and geographic characteristics and develop a list of communities that deserve the attention of policymakers and analysts.

Although Hurricane Katrina was in a league of its own, the structure of New Orleans's economy and society and the inadequacy of the government response explain the length of time it has taken for employment to recover. African Americans have disproportionately shouldered this cost. In Williamsburg, African Americans suffered the brunt of the storm, but evidence suggests that the losses were limited and short-lived. In both cases, we find that disparate racial impacts had less to do with the natural disasters' severity and more to do with the economic and social conditions prior to each disaster—including income inequality and, as Roland Anglin shows in his chapter, aging and outdated infrastructure and ineffective government.

What is the prognosis for addressing these three broad areas of vulnerability? In recent years, it does not seem as if analysts, advocates, and politicians who talk publicly about inequality are being charged with stoking class warfare. This is a positive development. But public budgets at all levels of government are tight, and the populace appears to have no appetite to finance the investments needed to address inequality, update aging public infrastructures, and reinvigorate government.

Simply put, to prepare for the future, budget priorities have to change. This dilemma reminds me of the old Fram oil filter commercial's tag line, "You can pay me now, or pay me later." Let it be hoped that we will not need another catastrophe of Katrina's or even Isabel's proportions to shift priorities.

NOTES

1. See, for example, "Issues and Insights after Hurricane Katrina," Urban Institute, October 4, 2005, http://www.urban.org/url.cfm?ID=900897.

2. William D. Nordhaus, "The Economics of Hurricanes in the United States," Yale University, Dept. of Economics, December 21, 2006, http://www.econ.yale.edu/~nordhaus/homepage/homepage.htm.

3. Jacob Vigdor, "The Katrina Effect: Was There a Bright Side to the Evacuation of Greater New Orleans?" National Bureau of Economic Research, working papers, 2007, http://www.nber.org/papers/w13022. Vigdor uses longitudinal data from Current Population Surveys conducted between 2004 and 2006 to estimate the net impact of Hurricane Katrina–related evacuation on various indicators of well-being. He concludes that there is little evidence to support the claim that poor, underemployed New Orleans residents were disadvantaged by their location in a relatively depressed region.

4. The Federal Emergency Management Agency's declaration data identifies two types of designations. A major disaster is defined as any natural catastrophe (including hurricanes, tornadoes, storms, high water, wind-driven water, tidal waves, tsunamis, earthquakes, volcanic eruptions, landslides, mudslides, snowstorms, or drought) or, regardless of cause, any fire, flood, or explosion, in any part of the United States, which in the determination of the president causes damage of sufficient severity and magnitude to warrant major disaster assistance. Federal funds become available to supplement the efforts and resources of states, local governments, and disaster relief organizations. An emergency is any event for which, in the determination of the president, federal assistance is needed to supplement state and local efforts and capabilities to save lives and to protect property and public health and safety, or to lessen or avert the threat of a catastrophe. The designation process is not straightforward. Rather, Rutherford Platt shows that a variety of factors, such as politics, influence designation. Rutherford H. Platt, *Disasters and Democracy: The Politics of Extreme Natural Events* (Washington, D.C.: Island Press, 1999).

5. The Current Employment Statistics national estimates for the month of September 2005, published on October 7, were the first to reflect the impact of Hurricane Katrina, subject to the collection and estimation issues discussed in this chapter. September estimates for state and metropolitan areas were first published on October 21. See the Bureau of Labor Statistics Web site for a detailed discussion of how the BLS modified its efforts to ensure greater reliability in the post-Katrina employment estimates, http://www.bls.gov/katrina/lausquestions.htm.

6. Texas, California, Florida, and Louisiana have the largest number of declarations. From 1953 to 2006, the number of declarations has risen. There are a variety of explanations for this upward trend. Some argue that global warming is the reason, but many communities have seen the percentage of their impervious surfaces increase over time, thus reducing the ability of an area's sewers, reservoirs, and rivers to handle a significant amount of rainfall.

7. Counties in Alabama and Mississippi also were officially designated disaster areas on August 29. Sharon P. Brown, Sandra L. Mason, and Richard B. Tiller, "The Effect of Hurricane Katrina on Employment and Unemployment," *Monthly Labor Review* 129, no. 8 (2006): 52–69.

8. U.S. Census Bureau, "Annual Estimates of the Population of Metropolitan and Micropolitan Statistical Areas: April 1, 2000 to July 1, 2008 (CBSA-EST2008-01)," March 19, 2009, http://www.census.gov/popest/metro/CBSA-est2008-annual.html.

9. U.S. Census Bureau, "2005–2007 American Community Survey," http://www.census.gov.

10. Author's calculation of data from the Bureau of Labor Statistics, "Current Employment Statistics (CES), Employment, Hours, and Earnings—State and Metro Area," http://www.bls.gov/data/#employment. Baton Rouge employment remained in the 340,000 range, and Shreveport employment remained in the 170,000 range.

11. The storm became a category 5 hurricane on September 11. It was the first category 5 hurricane in the Atlantic basin since Mitch in 1998. On September 12, Isabel reached its peak intensity with winds of 140 knots and a barometric pressure of 920 millibars.

12. See William M. Gray and Philip J. Klotzbach, "Summary of 2003 Atlantic Tropical Cyclone Activity and Verification of Author's Seasonal and Monthly Forecasts," Department of Atmospheric Science, Colorado State University (2003).

13. Nordhaus, "The Economics of Hurricanes in the United States."

14. Counties in West Virginia (September 23), Delaware (September 20 and 23), the District of Columbia (September 20), Maryland (September 19), and North Carolina (September 18) were also designated disaster areas. Hurricane Isabel destroyed many towns along the Chesapeake Bay and submerged downtown Baltimore and Annapolis in eight feet of water. See R. L. Ehrlich and J. W. Droneburg, "Preparing for an Emergency: Maryland State Agencies Continuity of Operations Planning for State Agencies," University of Maryland, Baltimore (2004). Estimates for Maryland are about $500 million of damage. Environment Maryland Research and Policy Center, *A Blueprint for Action: Policy Options to Reduce Maryland's Contribution to Global Warming*, 2007, http://cdn.publicinterestnetwork.org/assets/sDkxp5DPve8qPpp24giiXA/blueprint-for-action.pdf.

15. U.S. Census Bureau, "PCT112, Family Income in 1999," Census 2000 Summary File 4—Sample Data.

16. U.S. Census Bureau, "PCT76B, Poverty Status in 1999 of Related Children under 18 Years by Family Type by Age," Census 2000 Summary File 4—Sample Data.

17. Author's calculations of Bureau of Labor Statistics data. These data are obtained at http://www.bls.gov/data/#employment. Click on the Local Area Unemployment Statistics header, and choose a geographical area.

18. See, for example, Nordhaus, "The Economics of Hurricanes in the United States."

19. Ibid.

12

The Katrina Diaspora

Dislocation and the Reproduction of Segregation and Employment Inequality

NIKI T. DICKERSON

The natural disaster spawned by the 2005 hurricanes illuminated the poverty, unemployment, and low earnings of many black residents of the Gulf Coast. The people who fled their homes to other locales faced the life-altering question of whether to return to their former cities or make a new life in the places to which they evacuated. Was it better for black residents, particularly those who were not faring well in New Orleans before the hurricanes, to move on, or would similar dynamics of poverty and race reemerge and disadvantage Katrina evacuees in their new settings?[1]

To answer this question, I focus on economic and employment opportunities for evacuees. My analysis relies on the body of research connecting space and work as well as research on poverty and place (specifically the notion that economic and employment opportunities are linked to place).[2] My interest in the postdislocation employment and residential outcomes of displaced black Gulf Coast evacuees yields two central questions: (1) How did the dislocation and resettlement of Katrina and Rita evacuees improve, maintain, or worsen their employment and earnings outcomes? and (2) What mechanisms contributed to these outcomes?

Evidence for the arguments I make here come from employment data collected by the Current Population Survey (jointly produced by the U.S. Census Bureau and the Bureau of Labor Statistics), summary segregation and employment data on New Orleans, a large-scale survey of the shelter population in Houston (the metropolitan area receiving the largest displaced population) conducted by Rice University, interviews with volunteer organizations that assisted evacuees in other cities, and newspaper accounts. I find that race and class shape the opportunities of evacuees in new settings and contribute to the difficultly non-returnees have in obtaining employment and housing.

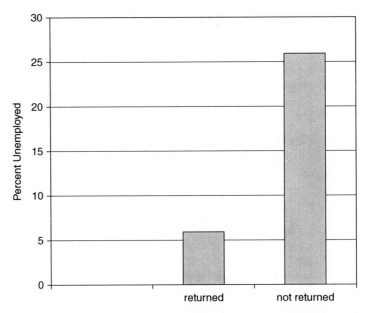

FIGURE 12.1. Percentage of Evacuees Unemployed, September 2006, by Dislocation Status.

Source: "The Labor Market Impact of Hurricane Katrina: An Overview," Bureau of Labor Statistics, *Monthly Labor Review Online* 129, no. 8 (August 2006): http://www.bls.gov/opub/mlr/2006/08/artifull/pdf.

What Happened? Relocation and Employment Outcomes

Approximately 2.2 million residents were displaced as a result of Hurricanes Katrina and Rita.[3] Of evacuees relocated by the Federal Emergency Management Agency (FEMA), 61.6 percent went to Texas and 27.0 percent went to Louisiana.[4] The metropolitan area of Houston, Texas, received the largest share of evacuees, estimated at between 100,000 and 160,000. A Rice University research team surveyed 1,081 of these displaced people and found that 69 percent intended to stay in Houston. In Houston, and other metropolitan areas, evacuees are less likely to be employed and, if employed, earn less on average than those who have returned.[5]

Figure 12.1 shows the dislocation status and employment outcomes for the Katrina evacuees. A year after the hurricane, the unemployment rate of displaced residents who had returned to their homes was 5.9 percent, whereas for those who had not yet returned, the unemployment rate was 25.6 percent.[6]

Figure 12.2 reveals that black evacuees were five times more likely to be unemployed than white evacuees. Because the federal government does not consider a person who is unemployed for over a year to be "actively looking for work," and therefore does not count these workers as part of the labor force,

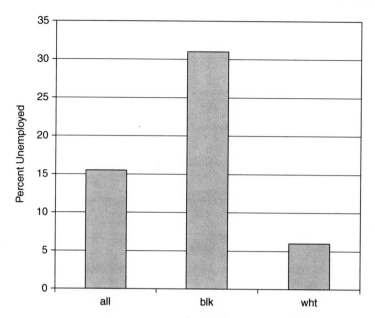

FIGURE 12.2. Percentage of Evacuees Unemployed, October 2005–June 2006.

Source: Bureau of Labor Statistics, "The Labor Market Impact of Hurricane Katrina: An Overview," *Monthly Labor Review Online* 129, no. 8 (August 2006): http://www.bls.gov/opub/mlr/2006/08/artıfull.pdf.

these figures may undercount the unemployed. Furthermore, because only residential homes are surveyed, these data do not capture the experiences of evacuees living in hotels or shelters. These two factors very likely led to a significant undercount of black evacuees, who were more likely than white evacuees to reside in shelters and experience long-term unemployment.

Figure 12.3 shows the unemployment rate for each group of evacuees (those who had returned home versus those who had not) on a monthly basis. The rate of unemployment seems to drop fairly rapidly for non-returnees in this sample. Non-returnees were presumably being slowly absorbed into the host metropolitan labor markets, but they might also have been dropping out of the formal labor market altogether, as figure 12.4 suggests. Figure 12.4 shows the percentage of evacuees employed, by dislocation status. While 58 percent of those who returned were employed a year after Katrina, only 41 percent of those who relocated were employed.

Non-returnees experienced a deterioration of both their employment status and earnings. Prior to their displacement, half of the employed respondents now in Houston reported earnings of less than $15,000 a year in the Rice survey. However, a year later their average income picture deteriorated: the percentage earning below $15,000 a year went from 44 percent to 74 percent, and those

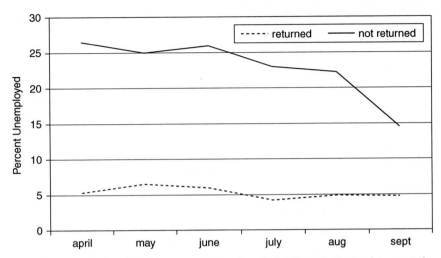

FIGURE 12.3. Percentage of Evacuees Unemployed, April 2006–September 2006, by Dislocation Status.

Source: Bureau of Labor Statistics, Employment Status Information on Hurricane Katrina Evacuees: http://www.bls.gov/katrina/empstatusinfo.htm; for 2006, http://www.bls.gov/katrina/200604status.htm

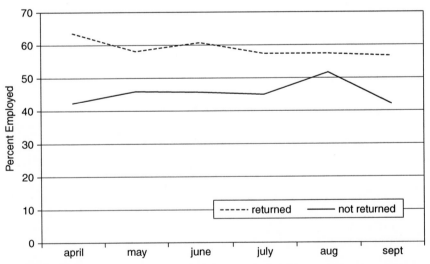

FIGURE 12.4. Percentage of Evacuees Employed, April 2006–September 2006, by Dislocation Status.

Source: Bureau of Labor Statistics, Employment Status Information on Hurricane Katrina Evacuees: http://www.bls.gov/katrina/empstatusinfo.htm; for 2006, http://www.bls.gov/katrina/200604status.htm

earning above $25,000 shrank. The percentage unemployed was more than two and a half times greater, growing from 27 percent to 70 percent (before the hurricane 66 percent were employed).[7] A survey of the ninety thousand evacuees in Houston's free housing program found that only 20 percent were employed.[8]

Recipe for Failure: Metropolitan Segregation and Employment Inequality

After touring one of the evacuation centers, Barbara Bush, former First Lady and mother of then President Bush, noted that because many of the people there were underprivileged, "this is working out well for them." Bush was correct that many of the displaced were "underprivileged." However, whether things would be "working out well for them" is not disconnected from their pre-storm problems. In other words, the socioeconomic status and employment situation of the evacuees before their displacement condition their postdisplacement outcomes.

The larger story of race and exclusion reflected by inferior local labor markets, social networks, and, ultimately, less wealth for black families, can help explain both preexisting racial disparities and those that emerged after Katrina. Social scientists contend that the link between social isolation and joblessness is the primary cause of ongoing inequality.[9] Residential segregation facilitates the unequal distribution of resources: access to jobs, quality schooling, productive job information networks, and transportation.[10] Segregation matters because resources are unevenly distributed across neighborhoods.

Residential segregation limits the black population's access to social and economic resources. It thereby depresses black employment rates and earnings.[11] Contemporary U.S. residential segregation levels are only moderately lower than during the Jim Crow era. Segregation is an exceptionally resilient structure that creates and maintains inequality. In urban labor markets, racial segregation within a city equals economic and social isolation for black communities, which, in turn, leads to employment difficulties.

Before the 2005 hurricanes, New Orleans was a highly segregated city marked by high concentrations of poverty. New Orleans, however, was not always a segregated city. Although heavily stratified by race and class, New Orleans neighborhoods were racially integrated throughout much of its history. In the 1950s, all-white and all-black neighborhoods began to form. As noted in the Brookings Institution report, "New Orleans after the Storm," "it wasn't until the 1960s and 1970s that New Orleans and other Southern cities started to see the hyper-segregation of Northern cities such as Chicago and Detroit."[12] While black/white segregation declined modestly in most cities between 1990 and 2000, not only did segregation increase in New Orleans, but the city witnessed one of the ten largest increases in the nation.[13] Metropolitan New Orleans's dissimilarity score was 69 (over 60 is considered highly segregated) at the neighborhood level, but that segregation was even more extreme than the number indicates. Several neighborhoods, like the Lower Ninth Ward, were almost 100 percent nonwhite. Furthermore, these minority neighborhoods were clustered in the midcity areas and the eastern half of the city.[14]

Because local labor markets limit individuals' employment opportunities, the characteristics of their local social and geographic space constrain their choices before and after displacement.[15] The supply of and demand for workers in a local labor market affect their likelihood of obtaining employment, and the quality of employment they can obtain. In New Orleans, employment was concentrated in low-wage service and tourist industries. The higher-wage industries in New Orleans, such as shipping and oil extraction, employed relatively few workers.[16] Not surprisingly, New Orleans had high levels of unemployment and below-average earnings compared with other large metropolitan areas. The egregiously high black unemployment rate in New Orleans, which was two-thirds black, was 20 percent higher than the national unemployment rate of all black workers.[17] This situation underscores the idea that blacks, in urban labor markets, represent a surplus supply of labor and are poorly integrated into the workforce. In most urban labor markets blacks have a weak attachment to their local economy.

Social scientists have also discovered the importance of social networks in finding employment. The quality of those in an individual's network determines how useful those associations are in providing information about jobs. For example, the job networks literature has demonstrated that blacks who use people in their network to find information about jobs end up with worse job outcomes than those who go outside of their immediate networks; the opposite is true for white job seekers.[18] This research speaks to the quality of blacks' and whites' networks. Each group replicates the employment outcomes of people in their network, and because whites on average have better jobs than blacks, black networks tend to yield worse results. Social networks—friends, family, and associates who provide information, in-kind support, access, referrals, and other resources—help people establish themselves in new cities.

Before the hurricanes of 2005 struck, many residents of New Orleans, particularly those in flood-prone areas, were economically vulnerable. National racial differences in wealth (savings, assets, etc.) are even starker than those in income; on average blacks have only 10 percent the wealth of whites.[19] Wealth refers to accumulated resources that people can draw on during times of crisis. After the hurricanes, in a new city, evacuees were bereft of the resources needed to find work, commute to work efficiently, and pay for market-rate housing within reasonable access to job-dense areas of the city.

After the Storm: Relocation Mechanisms and the Reconstitution of Inequality

Many relocation schemes reproduced previous inequalities. The mechanisms that came into play during relocation may explain the difficulty black evacuees have had in the resettlement process. In new cities, Katrina evacuees faced blatant housing discrimination and racial steering, which led to social and economic isolation, exacerbated by a break up of social networks and a lack of transportation.

The shelters to which many evacuees were relocated (in many cases not by choice) were often located in isolated areas of the city: the "black" side of town (in the case of San Antonio) or in predominantly black areas of the city (North Philadelphia), and near air force bases, which are typically located on the outskirts of cities where land is cheaper (San Antonio). In Philadelphia, initially some temporary shelters were located near the economically vibrant center city. However, the only long-term shelter where evacuees were housed was located in a predominantly black area of the city where jobs are scarce and poverty is high. In Philadelphia, city agencies that coordinated permanent housing searches for evacuees showed people public housing in Germantown, South and West Philly, and Fairmount Park—most of which are predominantly black neighborhoods. An analysis of the counties in Atlanta and Houston where a substantial number of evacuees relocated revealed that these areas have higher concentrations of minority residents and single mothers, and lower incomes than other counties.[20]

Early decisions focused on the most immediate and pressing needs—food, water, shelter—and thus, decisions were made quickly. An aid worker reported that shelters in San Antonio were places of chaos: "There were a thousand people in one room; there was fighting. Our primary concern was to get people out of the shelter as soon as we could."[21] However, quick, short-term decisions often have long-term consequences, as evacuees' initial placement determined where their eventual housing and employment search began.

Housing searches to find a better location nearer jobs or transportation ran into problems. Reports of housing discrimination in the Gulf region and U.S. metropolitan areas specifically targeted at black Katrina evacuees intensified barriers for black evacuees trying to reestablish themselves. After receiving complaints of discrimination, the national Fair Housing Alliance conducted controlled audits to test for discrimination. Matched pairs of black and white potential renters were sent to obtain housing. Out of sixty-five audits, there were forty-three (66 percent) in which blacks were discriminated against and/or white renters were favored. In some of these cases, black and white renters were given different information about the availability of rental units. Rental agents informed black renters that no units were available soon after telling white callers that there were. In other cases, black renters were less likely to have their phone calls returned. Landlords or rental agencies offered useful information to white callers, lied to black renters requesting information ("our computer is down"), quoted higher prices/deposits to blacks, offered special discounts and inducements for white renters, and waived security deposits for whites and not for blacks. In one case, a black renter was informed that income requirements were in effect, whereas the follow-up white renter was not told this. These trends in housing discrimination existed well *before* the hurricanes and reemerged as a significant obstacle for blacks who attempted to relocate.[22]

Researchers did not need to go far to find evidence of individual-level discrimination. As private households opened their homes to evacuees via Internet postings, racial preference and discrimination became evident again. Although the majority of postings did not mention a racial preference, those that did were explicit:

"As a white couple, we would be looking for a white mother and baby"

"We would prefer a white Christian couple"

"Not racist, but white only"[23]

Blocked out of housing in mainstream areas, blacks are pushed to areas of least resistance, that is, predominantly black neighborhoods, which effectively re-create the situations they left. Housing discrimination and resulting segregation amplifies the challenges they face finding work.[24]

More generally, reports of general discrimination and hostility toward evacuees in places with particularly large evacuee populations, Houston in particular, create difficulty for all evacuees. A stigma associated with evacuees made it hard even for the highly skilled to find work, particularly at their previous wage levels.[25] "[Houston] is different from New Orleans as far as opportunity, but they don't want to open it up to people from Louisiana," said Alphonso Thomas, a thirty-four-year-old evacuee in Houston. "Over 90 percent of the people here are either suicidal or hopeless."[26] The Rice survey of Houston evacuees reports high levels of psychological distress as well.

Complicating matters further, there was little coordination among FEMA, municipal agencies, and civic organizations providing support to evacuees. FEMA's deadlines of support mandated that assistance to help evacuees recover was temporary. Thus, FEMA support simply ended after a period of time without consideration of the evacuees' ability to support themselves. Some shelters closed even though some evacuees still remained; they were presumably turned out to fend for themselves, and many are likely now homeless. There is little evidence that there was guidance in finding employment in cities that were completely foreign to the newly arrived job-seekers. Furthermore, evacuees in the Rice study report that they have not been able to establish the social networks critical to job success.[27]

Evacuees interviewed spoke of going to new cities and not knowing the lay of the land or having transportation to look for jobs. "People didn't have anything," an aid worker told me. Sprawling southern cities, such as Atlanta and Houston, make cars a necessity rather than a luxury. Evacuees in Houston and Atlanta cite a lack of transportation as a chief problem, just as it was for residents in the storm area when it hit.[28] In San Antonio, after evacuees were placed in permanent housing, they were offered no employment assistance or counseling. "[We] pretty much left them alone."[29] There was little to no long-term follow through from FEMA, private aid organizations, or city agencies.

Lack of income was not the only problem for many black evacuees. An aid worker reported, "People came with nothing. They were close to abject poverty, without hope, and had a staunch attitude of not wanting to return."[30] Many left behind vital personal documents in their harried escape from the hurricanes: documents that are essential to procuring essential services, benefits, and jobs. The wide disparities in wealth (savings, assets, etc.) across race became a crucial factor as evacuees struggled to regain their financial footing. As William Rodgers explains in his chapter, reserve assets are critical, as they determine one's ability to make the transition to another means of support. Those who fled to families' homes are better off than those whose only choice was to seek public shelters, particularly those who left before the storms hit rather than after.

While many of the evacuees had poor educational backgrounds, interviews reveal that even educated and skilled evacuees faced difficulties reestablishing their previous earnings. Reports of teachers working as security guards or of an experienced forklift operator being offered only entry-level positions at $6 an hour represent the extent of employment problems for the displaced.[31] For some professional workers, certification requirements are a stumbling block. Because the qualification criteria for some occupations differ from state to state, those who had previously worked as teachers or nurses must recertify, a costly and cumbersome barrier.[32] Some report not being able to recertify and thus are unable to work in their previous occupations. If unchecked, these mechanisms will assure that previous inequalities are reestablished.

Conclusion and Policy Recommendations

Similar social and economic processes are replicating the pre-storm patterns of inequality. Solutions to reduce the isolation that results from residential segregation are necessary to address the poor employment outcomes for storm evacuees. If the political will to dismantle underlying structures does not come to the fore, and we, as a society, employ only superficial, Band-aid changes, larger social and economic forces will reduce recovery efforts to little more than a minor reshuffling of disenfranchised black people. As these people slowly reconstitute their prior socioeconomic standing, we will have effectively restored the racial structure so endemic to U.S. society. Hence, we will have preserved both the patterns of racial inequality and left exposed for the next disaster the same patterns of vulnerability.

Instead, we must begin with the realization that poverty is a structural problem and not an individual one. In other words, public policy and collective solutions will be necessary. Some possible solutions would be the enforcement of fair housing laws to combat housing discrimination, construction of public housing in neighborhoods with access to jobs, expanded social services that include job training and counseling, more public transportation, and living-wage laws. This is by no means an exhaustive or definitive list of the solutions to poverty, but it provides a place to start the conversation.

NOTES

1. Xavier de Souza Briggs, "After Katrina: Rebuilding Places and Lives," *City and Community* 5, no. 2 (2006): 119–128.

2. Ibid.

3. Louisiana Recovery Authority, "Hurricane Katrina Anniversary Data for Louisiana," http://www.lra.louisiana.gov/assets/docs/searchable/LouisianaKatrinaAnniversary Data082206.pdf.

4. Federal Emergency Management Agency, "Hurricane Katrina Response and Recovery Update," September 4, 2005, http://www.fema.gov/news/newsrelease.fema?id=18602.

5. Rick K. Wilson and Robert M. Stein, "Katrina Evacuees in Houston: One-Year Out," Rice University, Division of Social Sciences, September 8, 2006, http://brl.rice.edu/katrina/white_papers/white_paper_9_8_06.pdf.

6. "Hurricane Katrina Evacuees, September 2006," Bureau of Labor Statistics, http://www.bls.gov/katrina/200609status.htm.

7. Wilson and Stein, "Katrina Evacuees in Houston."

8. Shaila Dewan, "Storm's Escape Routes: One Forced, One Chosen," *New York Times*, August 24, 2006, sec. A.

9. For example, see Charles Tilly and Christopher Tilly, *Work under Capitalism* (Boulder, Colo.: Westview Press, 1998); James R. Elliott, "Social Isolation and Labor Market Insulation: Network and Neighborhood Effects on Less-Educated Urban Workers," *Sociological Quarterly* 40, no. 2 (1999): 199–216.

10. Niki Dickerson, "Black Employment, Segregation, and the Social Organization of Metropolitan Labor Markets," *Economic Geography* 83, no. 3 (2007): 283–307.

11. David M. Cutler and Edward L. Glaeser, "Are Ghettos Good or Bad?" *Quarterly Journal of Economics* 112, no. 3 (1997): 827–872.

12. Brookings Institution, "New Orleans after the Storm: Lessons from the Past, a Plan for the Future," 2005, http://www.brookings.edu/reports/2005/10metropolitanpolicy.aspx.

13. William Frey and Dowell Myers, "Racial Segregation in U.S. Metropolitan Areas and Cities, 1990–2000: Patterns, Trends, and Explanations," Population Studies Center Research Report No. 05–573 (Ann Arbor: University of Michigan, 2005).

14. Brookings Institution, "New Orleans after the Storm," 5–6.

15. Leslie McCall, "Sources of Racial Wage Inequality in Urban Labor Markets: Racial, Ethnic, and Gender Differences," *American Sociological Review* 66 no. 3 (2001): 520–541.

16. Brookings Institution, "New Orleans after the Storm."

17. Harry Holzer and Robert I. Lerman, "Employment Issues and Challenges in Post-Katrina New Orleans," Urban Institute, http://www.urban.org/url.cfm?ID=90092.

18. Gary Green, Leann Tigges, and Daniel Diaz, "Racial and Ethnic Differences in Job Search Strategies in Atlanta, Boston, and Los Angeles," *Social Science Quarterly* 80, no. 2 (1999): 263–278.

19. Thomas M. Shapiro and Jessica L. Kenty-Drane, "The Racial Wealth Gap," in *African Americans in the U.S. Economy*, ed. Cecilia A. Conrad, John Whitehead, Patrick Mason, and James Stewart, 175–181 (Lanham, Md.: Rowman and Littlefield, 2005).

20. Jason DeParle, "Katrina's Tide Carries Many to Hopeful Shores," *New York Times*, April 23, 2006, sec. I.

21. Volunteer worker, telephone interview by author, September 2006.

22. Douglas S. Massey and Garvey Lundy, "The Use of Black English and Racial Discrimination in Urban Housing Markets," *Urban Affairs Review* 36, no. 4 (2001): 452–470.

23. Ads posted on Katrinahousing.org, documented in "Greater New Orleans Fair Housing Action Center," draft congressional testimony (Housing Subcommittee on Housing and Equal Opportunity), February 28, 2006, http://www.gofairhousing.org/pdfs/2-28-06testimonyperry.pdf.

24. Dickerson, "Black Employment, Segregation, and the Social Organization of Metropolitan Labor Markets."

25. Ricard Wolf, "Evacuee Benefits Differ by State," *USA Today*, October 10, 2005.

26. Thomas quoted in Dewan, "Storm's Escape Routes."

27. Wilson and Stein, "Katrina Evacuees in Houston."

28. Dewan, "Storm's Escape Routes."

29. Volunteer worker, telephone interview by author, September 2006.

30. Ibid.

31. Dewan, "Storm's Escape Routes."

32. Ibid.

PART FOUR

Tragedy, Recovery, and Myth

13

Katrina and the Myth of Self-Sufficiency

DAVID DANTE TROUTT

I saw the deaths and was outraged. I felt the delays and started a book.[1] A year later, I went on the radio to talk about it. That's when "Jay" from St. Paul called in to make Katrina into the myth of self-reliance. I had just said something about how, a year into our 9/11-like sympathy and collective frustration, we were all "these people" in New Orleans. Jay's initial delivery stuttered with obvious exasperation. "I couldn't disagree more," he began. "It seems to me that these people took no responsibility for themselves. If this happened in the Twin Cities . . . the people that *I* know would have gotten out. I don't know *anybody* that doesn't have a car, or that doesn't have the means to get somewhere. So, to say that we're like these people is so far from . . ." Then he concluded, "I don't think that the residents of New Orleans took enough responsibility on themselves."[2]

I was grateful for Jay's call. I've been rebutting him ever since, even though the conversation continues to be one-sided—a direct contradiction to the promised debate on Katrina, race, and class that the contributors to *After the Storm*, and those writing in this volume, want to advance. There are many ways to talk about the continuing meanings of Hurricane Katrina. It was and is a colossal failure of government, an indictment of federal disaster relief, a travesty of engineering. It was and is a cumulative environmental tragedy, a belated reminder of our fragility against nature. It was and is the single largest public health debacle for the many thousands gone or gone off to struggle—with the heavy baggage of profound psychological trauma weighing on them—in unfamiliar, sometimes hostile places. The writers in this collection are keen to all of these dimensions, speaking elegantly and constructively about the remote possibility of transformation coming from this. Race and class are always implicated in these analyses; as a colleague of mine teaches, why they were poor had so much to do with why the survivors were black and why they were black says so much about why they were poor.

But the trouble always seems to be reaching Jay in St. Paul, consumed as he is—and he is not alone—with boiling this down to self-sufficiency. Our fleeting radio encounter not only prevents us from a dialogue, I also cannot see him. So, I only guess that he is white, approaching middle age like me, politically moderate, educated (he listens to National Public Radio), and lives comfortably in a stable, middle-class neighborhood that is almost all white, or at least hardly black. (I do not personally know the area except to have managed somehow to make not one but two white male best friends from Minneapolis.) It would help if I could put him in a suburb, but that he is middle class and probably lives in a racially segregated environment is enough.

I want to talk to him first about segregation's effect on self-sufficiency, both for its victims and its beneficiaries. Then I want to talk about localism, the legal brand name for his beliefs about forcing self-sufficiency on people deemed—by his criticism—the authors of their own misery. Ultimately, we would have a complex conversation about metropolitan interdependency and how we are running out of the known world. But nothing happens until we clear up this notion of the car.

A car, after all, is the opening measure in some American ballad of freedom that plays in Jay's head. Having one is a mark of citizenship and personal responsibility. Not having one seems derelict to him, the unreasonable denial of a necessity. I understand. I too see car commercials, images of reasonable-looking people at car dealerships getting sound information from caring, smiling salesmen, light touching between them, obvious affinity on both sides. Or I drive along a well-crafted highway, past new subdivisions and model homes, until I pass the Auto Mall (or whatever it's called where you live), with a dozen gleaming dealerships in a row on both sides of the road, distinguishable only by the particular logo in the center of the box-top buildings, cars like dream boats or breakfast cereal, lined up in aisles that await you. It is a ritual of middle-class life. It will happen again and again in that way every couple of years at the lease's end. (Only the gas mileage will stay the same.)

Yet it has absolutely nothing to do with the imagined cars of the kind of dark brown, poor people whom Jay thought should have cars in New Orleans. Instead, those cars are "jalopies," rightfully stopped by the police. They are the irresponsibly "tricked out" pimp rides of a ghetto fascination with rims, donuts, and drive-by shootings. They are the pink Cadillacs of "welfare queens" a political generation ago. They are the luxurious butts of a thousand racial jokes about vulgar excess, even if—like reports of raped babies, Superdome gang attacks, and rooftop storm survivors shooting at rescue helicopters—they are untrue.

What I suspect Jay has in mind is a form of automotive Americana, moving briskly from self-sacrificing work to cathedrals of consumption, which makes it extremely hard to see the Other when she waits desperately for a place at the desk where the social contract is reexecuted daily. Not just because she couldn't arrive by car, like so many in New Orleans. But because she lives a segregated life in the central city margins of a metropolitan economy that favors certain suburban quarters above all others. I have tried to read the evidence differently, but there is no more accurate way. Not only does "she" lack a seat at the table when the social contract is renegotiated, but she simply has no car. Thirty percent of New Orleans had no car that day;[3] unfortunately, many of those without cars tended to live near each other. Or together, and one was tied to a respirator or had dialysis treatment in the morning or was mostly bedridden after a stroke two years ago. And even if the old car worked, they had no place to go. They could not afford a hotel. They could not find one that was not already filled with evacuees. For America, the poor are mostly a blur; the fuzzy indiscernible images only coalesce into prepackaged stereotypes. When America does slow down to take a look, all we can say is "this is not America" and move on.

No, Jay cannot see her. He does not see them. He has neither known nor imagined knowing "these people" for long. I offer only possible facts, informed speculations at best. Jay's comments suggest that he is past facts and well into frames of reference that dictate which facts matter.[4] And I further assume that Jay does not live in one of those quarters where she and other survivors once lived, that he is merely middle class, and therefore that he may be unaware of the Katrina-size threat to his American dreams as a result of profoundly anti-majoritarian rules of localism that promote blind spots—to segregation, to sprawl, to environmental degradation, to declining suburbs, and to grossly inequitable cross-subsidization of the statewide fisc.[5] In the end, Jay is lucky. He will never be her, whatever his fate, because even the worst imaginable will not arise with the complicity of structural racism. Katrina reveals, however, that luck runs out while interdependency reigns.

Two Forms of Americanization in New Orleans

The first form of "Americanization," as Arnold Hirsch uses the term, began in New Orleans.[6] Social constructions of race had not always capitulated so easily to a black-white binary, especially in such a polyglot economic hub where they would have to be wrestled from ethnic meanings. Generations before Jay could ignore his status as a white person—if he is a white person—and simply speak for the norm, whites in New Orleans were not just white but Creole (Spanish or French) or Irish or German or Italian. By the early nineteenth century, the "American" (Yankee Protestant) presence had grown in number and influence, along with a deep distaste for racial mixing. That is, there were different ways of being white, just as there were ethnic differences among "blacks." Over time, a bloody civil war and the backlash of Reconstruction, white American impatience with racial pluralism yielded a familiar binary: offering whiteness for some and denying choice to the black remainder. There is more to this narrative, of course, but the basic outlines of a binary capitulation hold. A complex New Orleans gave in to facile American constructions of racial identity.

In the second form of Americanization, New Orleans ceded its earth to Jim Crow. After the Civil War, the impassable landscape and complicit climate made the city a model of urban planning on a high-ground grid. Racial tension, population growth, and technology, however, led to expansion into the swamps, lakefront, and eventually beyond. Pumps and canals allowed horizontal growth. But the human densities were lost, and the racial proximities of a local culture accustomed to sharing space were exchanged for separation. Jim Crow segregation formalized spatial arrangements in New Orleans in patterns more common to other large American cities. There is a lot about New Orleans that is unique, but its racial exceptionalism is belied by its racial geography.

Localism Ascendant

Especially with the postwar advent of suburbanization, the two-sided story of the country's romantic, though inequitable march to suburbia is well known. It mostly reflects the triumph—politically, economically, and geographically—of a way of life, an American Dream, complete with single-family detached homes, bucolic settings, and a paramount concern for the welfare of one's own family in all things. When that idealized story of the dream was complicated by the reality of state-sponsored racial and economic discrimination in the provision of mortgages or the lengthy history of private discrimination by the real estate, banking, and insurance industries—that is, when the American Dream ran headlong into the Rev. Martin Luther King Jr.'s even more idealized dream of racial equality, a third "triumph" was embraced: color-blind innocence. This could only occur with the advent of race-neutral rules, which localism offered.

By "localism" I refer to the term local government law scholars ascribe to the theory of local sovereignty or municipal self-determination. The idea fit the suburban model well. Developing suburbs grew up around the economic concern for stable or rising property values as much as for a sense of safety, community, and aesthetic appeal. Citizen residents grew up as much in love with suburban ideals as in contempt for urban realities. The rules of local control over land use enabled democratically elected zoning boards, for instance, to determine optimal lot sizes, maintain a healthy tax base, and welcome only certain types of business traffic. Local control of property tax revenues facilitated the pursuit of localized educational priorities, one of the most important reasons ours has become a suburbanized nation. That and of course cars.

The problem with localism, I would tell Jay, is that it is also a thinly disguised successor to racial segregation. By using economic discrimination as a proxy for race, it has worked almost as well as Jim Crow. It will be more durable over time, because the Supreme Court in the 1970s shielded it from constitutional attack with a nearly impenetrable jurisprudential edifice. In a handful of critical cases, the high court followed the lead of state courts and sanctioned the exclusionary effects of color-blind processes that suburbs had used to define their members and their outsiders;[7] to deny the construction of multifamily housing and public housing projects;[8] to ignore the negative externalities caused by defensive zoning rules;[9] to maintain huge disparities in public school funding between rich and poor districts;[10] and to relieve themselves of participation in interjurisdictional remedies for segregated schools.[11] In this way, cultural localism—the impulse to exclude and to define oneself narrowly— was aided by legal localism, mainly because the rules at issue cleverly avoided the making of any racial distinctions whatsoever.

The distinctions with the clearest discriminatory impact were economic, but the consequences for the excluded followed clear racial patterns. In New Orleans, like many metropolitan areas of the country, suburban localism hastened its urban antithesis: ghettoization, the poverty-concentrating effects of white flight, suburban sprawl, segregation, and the fiscal fatigue of the central city. While federal and state law and policy aided the affordable development of localist suburbs through highway construction and mortgage programs, federal and state housing policies such as urban renewal and siting rules for public housing developments undermined cities. No city better illustrated these structural fissures than New Orleans, whose poverty, school failures, joblessness, murder rates, and increasing segregation were legendary long before Katrina.

Why would a nation struggling to desegregate adopt localism, a nominally race-neutral system with demonstrable segregative effects? I would argue there are at least five reasons, perhaps six. First, localism was especially attractive in the postwar period because of its underlying commitment to economic rationalism. In short, maximizing property values by excluding high densities makes practical fiscal sense. Second, localism was the perfect suburban paradigm for smallness, and smallness favors decentralization. Decentralization is precisely what we've gotten, as the fetishism of local control (and the amenities it can bring on a small scale) proliferates municipalities. Third and relatedly, localism fosters political fragmentation—but theoretically allows more political participation at more meaningful levels of government. Again, the more small units of government there are, the better for democracy. Fourth, localism has grown up in an environment of increased consumption. The segregative effects of local control and interlocal competition for "good tax ratables" is not easily questioned when it is subsumed in a commodity—the house, neighborhood, and schools buyers get for the purchase price. Finally, there is evidence that middle-class black people—the primary actors in non-gentrification-based integration—are skeptical about the benefits of living in predominantly white neighborhoods.[12]

A sixth reason may go to the heart of Jay's comments: localism is seen as somehow a product of, and as conducive to, fostering individual merit.[13] In its notions of a collective local sovereignty, it may also affirm the individual member's powerful right to belong. Membership is a meritocracy. Only those who earn membership participate in the local democracies that control enough resources to matter locally. The middle-class ideals underlying localism, therefore, embody the status and rewards of responsible citizenship.

I appreciate Jay's comments even if they confirm what I believe Katrina most represents. The first thing he means to make clear is that nobody should ever link him to anyone incapable of taking full responsibility for themselves. He checked me lest I attempt to close some human distance between him and his friends and the survivors in New Orleans. They are distinct, and their difference boils down to a matter of character, as personal responsibility always is. He also assured other listeners from the community of working car owners that such a nightmare will never happen to them. He has excluded the survivors from his locality, and he has thereby excluded the locality from the possibility of a fate like Katrina. And in the distinction Jay must make a rigid binary assertion, ultimately of a responsible "us" and an irresponsible "them." In the distancing, I see de facto segregation. In the impatient disbelief about the absence of a car, I hear the consumption. In one brief statement, Jay has asserted the twin pillars of Americanization from behind the color-blind safety of a localist mindset.

The Disconnected Self

Yet it is not clear to me who the self is in Jay's notion of "self-sufficiency." No case can be made for either self-sufficiency or interdependency without a clearer idea of the self in these conflicts (and it was bound to become a conflict). Obviously, Jay did not assert an empathic self, an especially Christian self, or a humanistic self. The self of his self-sufficiency has some of the self of the residents of Gretna, who cheered their police chief's decision to forcibly turn back survivors fleeing New Orleans as they were heading toward neighboring Jefferson Parish. It is also not the criminal self of nihilism after the storm, killing and stealing the half-built remains of survivors' efforts to come home still. It is not the shamed self of New Orleans public officials, indicted for bribes or other acts of aggrandizement just when the city most needed their leadership. Nor is it equal to the indomitable self of those survivors who slowly put it back together, month by month, a quiet determination racked by setbacks but steeled by a never-say-no-return commitment to the familiar. And hopefully, it is not the suicidal self of some Federal Emergency Management Agency (FEMA) trailer camps, whose utter isolation in a time of dislocation has led to constant crime, substance abuse, depression, and their fatal consequences—like some sick, government-sponsored ghetto experiment in miniature.[14]

But Jay's self probably includes the family, and that's a fair place to start. Self-sufficiency among family members in cities like New Orleans has taken a beating because of the thirty-to-fifty-year transfer of jobs, political power, and fiscal resources not only to the global labor economy, but to suburbia.[15] Poor populations in central cities are considerably weaker now than they might have been without the exodus of resources to areas only cars can reach. Self-sufficiency in New Orleans has been perniciously denied survivors by the incompetence of the federal rescue, FEMA, the Louisiana Road Home program, and a great many other mostly public but many private institutions. More than most of us, New Orleanians often define themselves in connection with their families, not merely as a single household loading up a sports utility vehicle. What self-sufficiency many families had—and it might have been substantial— was suspended indefinitely by the events, policies, and unexpected constraints following this far-too-predictable disaster.

For a self whose sense of reliance and sufficiency is bound up in connections to family, especially young children and older relatives, the marks of Katrina continue to be made years after the deluge. We are so much more than our mortgages and leases, and Katrina reminded us that when the stable familiarity of our lives is suddenly dashed from us, the anchors lift and we are mentally at sea. As Nancy Boyd-Franklin makes so poignantly clear in her chapter, a great many Katrina survivors experienced trauma sufficient to produce post-traumatic stress disorder. PTSD can be difficult to treat in stable communities with proper resources; imagine what it's like in relocation limbo. PTSD can produce anxiety attacks, depression, stifling fear, disorientation, inability to trust, and related physical ailments. Then, beyond those directly suffering from PTSD, there is the radius of mental disorders—those who suffer vicarious PTSD, those whose trauma was less immediate but has accumulated with disappointments over time, those for whom trauma has combined with other mental illness and become debilitating. Then there is everyone who must depend on those who are struggling with PTSD, perhaps badly, through violent rages, alcohol and substance abuse, overeating, and distraction.[16]

Of course, what Katrina threatened to reveal about hardship, community, and self-sufficiency in about five raw and agonizing days of news coverage has assumed its invisible form again. It is not just the invisibility of very poor urban lives amid struggle. It is our culture's unwillingness to stare for long or with sincere empathy at any struggle to achieve self-sufficiency against overwhelming circumstances. Much has produced this. But the idea of localism, I argue, is chief among the reasons. It is ironically a framework for citizen participation in a narrow community as much as for a self disconnected from nonmembers and who is therefore more willing to blame them for their own sorrows.

And in this I suspect that Jay is right. *We* are not Katrina's most visible victims. Most of us live in relatively stable, rationally planned neighborhoods, institutionally connected to some sense of community where, by mostly efficient leadership, a tax base worthy of political attention, and good economic luck, the many markets of support keep us safe from sudden death. Our friends have cars. Our streets don't flood. *We are Jay.*

Conclusion: Equitable Regionalism

Although we are like Jay in a material sense, conditioned in part by localist designs, it is unfortunate that some of us would take the occasion of other people's suffering to extol our own self-sufficiency. Perhaps that is the route to empathy, however, because our self-sufficiency is mythical. We do not stand on our own, because the computer will crash, someone will fail to hear us, or the car will not start. And when those risks do not materialize, we can only thank our lucky stars that we did enough of the right things to land in a place where the computer kept working, somebody was attentive, the car started (and the streets were passable). To keep luck out of the game, many of us watch carefully to make sure our middle-class amenities are not slipping into decline, that the walls of the gated fortress hold, that property values rise. Increasingly across American suburbs, however, those ideals are jeopardized by rising property taxes, declining infrastructure, health and housing costs that consume a disproportionate amount of our incomes, and jealousy for what the new subdivisions in farther out towns and cities offer.[7] So, many of us move. We follow businesses, which follow lower taxes, which follow fresh new allocations of highway, water, and sewer infrastructure revenues from a state treasury paid for by the rising taxes of where we lived before. This is sprawl. It is also the wasteful, antimajoritarian, leapfrogging destiny of localism under current local government law and public finance. It works for some but not for many, and it is paid for by all. Because we are running out of space, it will end eventually, ceded probably to another inequitable dynamic that lacks transparency.

Unless we reform rules of local sovereignty in such a way as to reallocate fiscal burdens across whole regions, we cannot expect declining suburbs and central cities to bear the load of service delivery to a diminishing tax base alone. They can't. Depending on where Jay lives, he may already be feeling this pinch. *Our* self-sufficiency, the self-sufficiency of good fortune and impermanent membership in semiprivate municipal clubs of a middle-class good life, is at risk because of the inherent inequities that consistently favor wealthier interests over others and force municipalities to compete *not* to lose. Cooperation is a more effective model. Economic integration is normatively superior and also more efficient. The white poor in America, for instance, do not live in the same degree of isolation as the black poor, and the white poor do not stay poor as long. Equitable regionalism, as I propose it, is a principle based on sharing across regions the burdens that localism concentrates, such as affordable housing, tax base revenues, and school financing. Properly configured, states may see that what is good for their poorest members is good for the middle class as well.

Remarkably, the final irony to show Jay is that there is only one place I know of that has passed comprehensive legislation embracing the principle of equitable regionalism. That would be his home state of Minnesota.

NOTES

1. David Dante Troutt, ed., *After the Storm: Black Intellectuals Explore the Meaning of Hurricane Katrina* (New York: New Press, 2006).

2. See "Exploring the Lessons of Katrina," *MPRnewsQ*, August 28, 2006, Minnesota Public Radio, http://minnesota.publicradio.org/display/web/2006/08/28/midmorning2.

3. Brookings Institution, "New Orleans after the Storm: Lessons from the Past, a Plan for the Future" (October 2005), 19, http://www.brookings.edu/reports/2005/10metropolitanpolicy.aspx.

4. The insight behind this distinction comes from a careful and instructive discussion by law professors Cheryl Harris and Devon Carbado in "Loot or Find: Fact or Frame?" in Troutt, *After the Storm*.

5. "Fisc" is an expression—usually modified by the word "public"—to describe what all taxpayers pay into.

6. See Arnold R. Hirsch, "Simply a Matter of Black and White: The Transformation of Race and Politics in Twentieth-Century New Orleans," in *Creole New Orleans: Race and Americanization*, ed. Arnold R. Hirsch and Joseph Logsdon, 262–320 (Baton Rouge: Louisiana State University Press, 1992).

7. *Village of Belle Terre v. Boraas*, 416 U.S. 1 (1974).

8. *Village of Arlington Heights v. Metropolitan Housing Development Corp.*, 429 U.S. 252 (1977).

9. *Warth v. Seldin*, 422 U.S. 490 (1975).

10. *San Antonio School Independent District v. Rodriguez*, 411 U.S. 1 (1973).

11. *Milliken v. Bradley*, 418 U.S. 717 (1974).

12. Sheryll D. Cashin, "Middle-Class Black Suburbs and the State of Integration: A Post-Integrationist Vision for Metropolitan America," *Cornell Law Review* 86 (2001): 729.

13. Others have made related points. See, e.g., Matthew D. Lassiter, *The Silent Majority: Suburban Politics in the Sunbelt South* (Princeton, N.J.: Princeton University Press, 2006), 28.

14. Alix Spiegel, "Stuck and Suicidal in a Post-Katrina Trailer Park," National Public Radio broadcast, August 8, 2007.

15. Brookings Institution, "New Orleans after the Storm," 11–12.

16. See, generally, American Psychological Association, "Tornadoes, Hurricanes and Children," 2005, http://www.apahelpcenter.org/articles/article.php?id=109; National Child Traumatic Stress Network, "What You Should Know about Hurricanes," http://www.nctsnet.org/nccts/nav.do?pid=typ_nd_hurr_desc; GAO, Health, Education, and Human Services Division, *Elementary School Children: Many Change Schools Frequently, Harming Their Education*, GAO Report to House of Representatives, February 1994, http://archive.gao.gov/t2pbat4/150724.pdf.

17. See David Rusk, *Inside Game/Outside Game: Winning Strategies for Saving Urban America* (Washington, D.C.: Brookings Institution, 1999); Myron Orfield, *Metropolitics: A Regional Agenda for Community and Stability* (Washington, D.C.: Brookings Institution, 1997).

14

Race, Vulnerability, and Recovery

KEITH WAILOO

KAREN M. O'NEILL

JEFFREY DOWD

As rescue helicopters hover overhead and media cameras roll, a group of young people, all African American, stand on the rooftop of a house, holding a sign, "Help us!" In the storm's aftermath, families huddle in the shadow of a highway overpass, seeking shelter beneath the road that might have led them, under different circumstances, to safety. In one of Katrina's more horrific images, a body floats face down in the water—graphic proof of the storm's wrath, the broken levees, the water's violent assault on the residents of New Orleans, and the failure of the city, the state, and the nation to protect its people. As shocking as these images of Katrina were, they have also begun to fade from American memory, receding year by year as the region attempts to recover after the physical destruction and psychological trauma.

This book is not merely an effort of historical recovery but an analysis of Katrina as a sentinel American event and its continuing reverberations in contemporary politics, culture, and public policy. As the essays in this volume show, the Hurricane Katrina disaster was an indictment of earlier and more silent Katrinas. Together they provide a critique of how policy by increment harms the weakest. They reveal how the persistence of separate and unequal transportation systems, and how the policies and unfulfilled promises of government affect the health and well-being of its citizens. Katrina also revealed a graphic breach in the social fabric—with bodies being discovered into the fall of 2005, and the funereal atmosphere around the iconic American city. With its many houses destroyed by the storm, its citizens dispersed, and its trauma radiating outward, New Orleans remains haunted by the perception that no one really cares and no one would truly want to live there again. But Katrina also signaled resilience for a city whose jazz roots and people evoked pain as well as hope and celebration in spite of the hand they had been dealt. A milestone event in American history, Katrina also opened a new public vista on the complexity of race and vulnerability. It offered the U.S. media a new lens for writing about disasters and race; it reframed the question of leadership, preparedness, and security in both private and public sectors; and yet (sadly) it became a force for replicating pre-storm inequalities in housing, labor, and economic opportunity—scattering the city's former residents far and wide. Looking back and looking ahead, the challenge remains how to translate these new insights on race, trauma, vulnerability, and opportunity in America into policies that address the nation's everyday Katrinas and that will also mitigate the impact of the next storm, whatever form it takes.

As most of us know, recovery poses an epic challenge. After the hurricane, the devastation resulted not only from the forces of nature but from underlying and long-standing sociohistorical forces. Nature alone could not account for the way Katrina's impact was felt across the region and the nation. President George W. Bush himself pointed to the historical roots of poverty as partially located in racial regimes of America's past. Yet for Bush, as for most Americans, that is where the discussion of racism in creating the Katrina disaster began and ended. For other Americans, however, Katrina required deeper scrutiny. In this volume, for example, Karen O'Neill analyzes Katrina as a story of environmental justice, viewing the long-standing North-South divide, in which national leaders made accommodations to southern elites and supported hierarchical (and most often racial) power structures, as essential to that story. Similarly, Mia Bay calls attention to the history of racial inequalities in transportation—to "invisible tethers" that have constrained the mobility of black Americans. Bay insists that our society needs to understand its role in shaping transportation inequities and must address how transportation perpetuates long-existing inequalities. More generally, this book argues, reinvention cannot happen without studying Katrina's imprint—that is, without characterizing accurately the city before Katrina, documenting comprehensively the loss, investigating extensively the tangled nature of vulnerability, and (only then) charting a wise course toward reinvention and a true recovery.

As we write nearly five years after the awful event, New Orleans has not returned to "normal," nor will it. Indeed, it remains unclear what a normal New Orleans will look like. The city will be rebuilding for decades to come. But more important for this study, the structural inequalities that created the city's vulnerabilities in 2005 are still present for residents who returned, and new vulnerabilities have emerged for residents who have fled permanently only to find lives of poverty in other locations. As Katrina fades from the public conversation, Americans risk descending back into a pre-Katrina state of blissful ignorance and denial about the very vulnerabilities that created the disaster. We delude ourselves if we believe that those vulnerabilities were unique to this storm or confined to New Orleans.

One cannot fully "recover" as a nation from Katrina without recalling the racialized nature of the trauma and without grappling with the historical complexities of race and racism in America. As Ann Fabian writes in her chapter, the unburied bodies that haunted us in media reports were mostly black bodies, and these images of death have fused with images of a city lost—in ways that can, for some, never be forgotten. It is clear that many African Americans will remember the events in particular ways, and that particular events will be foremost in their retellings. What happened at the bridge at Gretna, for example, when police turned back New Orleans residents fleeing the storm's aftermath, will long be remembered. Few policies can address that injury—a collective behavior that also was rooted in entrenched structural inequalities. How long people waited on their roofs for rescue will continue to be remembered, as well as the inadequate water and food in the Superdome. Even those not intimately familiar with the southern ritual of jazz funerals that Richard Mizelle describes can appreciate the indignity of people being denied a proper funeral in a depopulated city. The images of abandoned houses, which Evie Shockley describes, are likely to stay with us, signifying the constant threat for blacks that they may be displaced by faceless social forces, by real live antagonists, by floods or by fire, in a society that has historically left them only marginal room for living. Still, while Nancy Boyd-Franklin acknowledges that these tales are painful reminders of a tortured past, she also concludes that African Americans remain resilient—and hopeful about the city's and nation's recovery.

With this volume, we remember Katrina and honor those who suffer and who still suffer; but the essays also go much further—examining privilege as well, and looking closely at the web of beliefs, attitudes, practices, and policies that gave rise to the Katrina event and that cast a shadow over the process of rebuilding and starting over. There is still much to learn about, and from, Katrina—about how transportation failures, environmental risks, health vulnerabilities, and poverty continue to intersect today to put people into harm's way and, importantly, keep others safe. As legal scholar Martha Fineman has written, "vulnerability inquiry examines the ways in which societal resources are channeled to see if the result is to privilege and protect some while tolerating the disadvantage and vulnerability of others."[1] Thus, we must continually reexamine Katrina not only to recall the acute crisis in 2005 but also to understand the chronic recurring processes by which Americans address some vulnerabilities and yet ignore and forget others. We see Katrina as a case study of the problem of vulnerability and privilege and as an argument for why we should not wait for another major disaster to take action.

Reflecting on the complex structural origins of the Katrina debacle and the systemic vulnerabilities it reveals, it is easy to come away cynical. Attention to the "structural origins" of any event can seem to draw attention away from the human action (or inaction) that creates and maintains those vulnerabilities. But seeing that Katrina was produced by collective actions—by decisions, policies, and practices—far upstream of the events turns attention to how individuals, groups, and actions created the structures, which, in turn, produced what we saw in the aftermath of Hurricane Katrina. By refocusing not on the structures per se but on the collective actions and policies that created roads, homes, levees, and dialysis centers, we see this book as an invitation to rethink how privilege and vulnerability were made in the first place. Even as they work toward rebuilding and recovery, there is much that elected officials, policymakers, and citizens can learn by looking closely yet again at Katrina, at the faces of hope and despair in 2005, and at the long history of federal, state, and city policies that worked together to *produce* the problems of poverty and privilege that we now seek to solve.

NOTE

1. Martha Albertson Fineman, "The Vulnerable Subject: Anchoring Equality in the Human Condition," *Yale Journal of Law and Feminism* 20 (2008): 20–21.

NOTES ON CONTRIBUTORS

JOHN R. AIELLO is a professor of psychology at Rutgers University and contributes to the Graduate Program in the Industrial Relations and Human Resources Department. Jack has published more than sixty articles and book chapters and has given more than three hundred invited addresses at professional meetings and business organizations.

ROLAND ANGLIN is the director of the Initiative for Regional and Community Transformation (IRCT) at the Edward J. Bloustein School of Planning and Public Policy, Rutgers University. The IRCT is a national initiative whose mission is to support the transformation of marginalized communities and people through the production of relevant knowledge and public policy strategies.

MIA BAY is an associate professor at Rutgers University and the associate director of the Rutgers Center for Race and Ethnicity. She is the author of two books, *The White Image in the Black Mind: African-American Ideas of White People, 1830–1925* and *To Tell the Truth Freely: The Life of Ida B. Wells*.

NANCY BOYD-FRANKLIN is a professor in the Graduate School of Applied and Professional Psychology at Rutgers University. Her research addresses the treatment of African-American families. She has written numerous articles and chapters and five books, including *Black Families in Therapy: Understanding the African American Experience* and *Reaching Out in Family Therapy: Home-Based, School, and Community Interventions* with Dr. Brenna Bry.

NIKI T. DICKERSON is an assistant professor in the Department of Labor Studies at Rutgers University. She is concerned with how U.S. racial economic inequality is sustained. Her current work examines the impact of residential segregation on the race gap in unemployment and wages for blacks and Latinos in U.S. metropolitan areas.

JEFFREY DOWD is a doctoral candidate in the Sociology Department at Rutgers University. He served two years as a graduate assistant at the university's

Center for Race and Ethnicity. Jeff teaches courses on race relations, social problems, and minority groups. His research deals with racial inequality and public discourse.

ANN FABIAN is dean of humanities and teaches American studies and history at Rutgers University. She writes on the cultural history of the United States in the nineteenth century. Her books include studies of gambling, as well as personal narratives. Her new book, *Headhunting: Flatheads, Fijians, and America's Skull-Collecting Naturalists*, will be published in 2010.

RICHARD MIZELLE JR. is an assistant professor in the Department of History at Florida State University. His specialization is twentieth-century U.S. social and cultural history, with an emphasis on the history of race and health in America. His current research project examines the social and cultural dimensions of the Great Mississippi Flood of 1927.

KAREN M. O'NEILL is a sociologist and associate professor of human ecology at the School of Environmental and Behavioral Sciences, Rutgers University. She specializes in contention, inequality, and state power in the United States. O'Neill is author of *Rivers by Design: State Power and the Origins of U.S. Flood Control*.

WILLIAM M. RODGERS III is a professor at the Edward J. Bloustein School of Planning and Public Policy, Rutgers University, and chief economist at its John J. Heldrich Center for Workforce Development. His research examines issues in labor economics and the economics of social problems. His most recent book, *The Handbook on the Economics of Discrimination*, was selected by *Choice*, the review journal of the American Library Association, as an "Outstanding Academic Book" for 2006.

EVIE SHOCKLEY is an assistant professor in the Department of English at Rutgers University. Shockley's scholarly essays include "Buried Alive: Gothic Homelessness, Black Women's Sexuality, and (Living) Death in Ann Petry's *The Street*" and "The Horrors of Homelessness: Gothic Doubling in Kincaid's *Lucy* and Brontë's *Villette*," in *Jamaica Kincaid and Caribbean Double Crossings* (edited by Linda Lang-Peralta).

LYRA STEIN is currently a graduate student in the Rutgers psychology doctoral program. She graduated from Rutgers University majoring in biochemistry and psychology and then earned her graduate degree in neuroscience. Her interests include personality predictors of behavior, both in organizations and in virtual environments.

DAVID DANTE TROUTT is a professor of law and Justice John J. Francis Scholar at Rutgers Law School–Newark. In 2006, he edited a collection of essays titled *After the Storm: Black Intellectuals Explore the Meaning of Hurricane Katrina* and authored the lead essay, "Many Thousands Gone, Again."

KEITH WAILOO is Martin Luther King Jr. Professor of History at Rutgers University. He has written widely on issues of health, race, and history. He is the author of *Dying in the City of the Blues: Sickle Cell Anemia* and the *Politics of Race and Health* and coeditor of *A Death Retold: Jesica Santillan, the Bungled Transplant, and Paradoxes of Medical Citizenship.*

INDEX

African American churches, 37, 69–71, 79, 88–90, 94n58
African Americans, 2–5, 45, 54n4, 194; and dead bodies, 59–67; denied entry to Gretna, 4, 81–83, 103, 188, 194; and engineering the river, 10–16, 18; and gothic homelessness, 95–99, 101–111, 112n25; and health-care system, 36–37; as homeowners, 15, 71–72, 87, 107–110, 151n8; housing patterns of, 10–12, 14–16; and jazz funerals, 69–76; and Jim Crow laws, 15, 23, 84, 87, 173, 186; in Katrina diaspora, 2, 101, 111n9, 169–171, 173–177 (see also displacement; evacuees); labor market impact on, 154–155, 160–166, 161; migration of, 73, 76, 98, 101–102; and myth of self-sufficiency, 183, 185, 187; New Orleans as icon of culture, 3, 15, 69–76, 102, 139, 151n8; and psychological trauma, 78–87, 89–90, 90–91n3; and public- vs. private-sector preparedness, 138–140; resilience of, 71, 79, 87–89, 94n58; segregation of, 14–15, 22–24, 46, 82–85, 87, 90–91n3, 99, 154, 173–176, 186; small businesses of, 138–140; social networks of, 15–16, 73, 79–80, 88–89, 140, 174–175; spirituality of, 87–89, 94n58; stereotyping of, 25, 80–81, 87, 96, 98–99, 103, 105, 110; and transportation system, 22–30. See also Middle Passage; slavery
African diaspora of slavery, 2, 90–91n3
African religions, 60, 65, 94n58
After the Storm (Troutt), 183
AIDS, 37–38
Aiello, John R., 3, 5, **135–153**, 197
Altman, Drew, 85–86
American Community Survey (2005), 161
American Society of Civil Engineers, 127
Amtrak, 29–30
Anglin, Roland, 2, 4, 11, 16, 31, **45–55**, 128, 166, 197
animal rescue, 146–147
Armstrong, Louis, 72, 74, 76
Army Corps of Engineers, U.S., 11–14, 16–17, 49
Astrodome (Houston), 40, 96, 108
attics, 14, 60–61, 66
automobiles, 16, 24–27, 29, 31, 64, 90–91n3, 129–130, 148, 163, 177; economics of

ownership, 25–27, 32n17; and myth of self-sufficiency, 3, 183–186, 188–190; parking for, 26–27, 32n17. *See also* transportation system
Ayres, Ian, 26

Baker, Richard H., 110
banks, 24, 135–137, 139–140, 144
Banks, Gralen B., 76, 77n20, 103–104
Bay, Mia, 2–4, 16, **21–33**, 52, 96, 193, 197
Beloved (Morrison), 100
Benga, Ota, 107, 113n33
Berry, Jason, 70
Biagi, George, 123
Bible, 73, 87
Billingsley, Andrew, 89
bin Laden, Osama, 34
Blanco, Kathleen, 62
Block, Melissa, 72
Body Worlds (exhibition), 59
Bonnie (hurricane), 121
Booth, William, 124
Border Patrol, 103
Borgne, Lake, 16
Boyd-Franklin, Nancy, 2, 4, **78–94**, 189, 194, 197
brass bands, 69–71
Brontë, Charlotte, 100
Brookings Institution, 173
Brown v. Board of Education, 23, 31
Bruce, Frank, 124
Burton, Linda, 78
buses. *See* transportation system
Bush, Barbara, 96, 98, 108, 173
Bush, George W., 1, 4, 6, 50, 63–64, 66, 193; and loopholes for federal contracts, 140; post-Katrina media coverage of, 124–127
businesses, 14, 16, 30, 53, 122; and gothic homelessness, 97, 108, 113n42; minority businesses, 138–140; and public- vs. private-sector preparedness, 135–150; small businesses, 135–141, 144–148, 150. *See also* private sector
Butts, Hugh F., 93n39

canals, 9, 14–16, 36
Carter, Karen, 103
Castle of Otranto, The (Walpole), 99–100
Catholicism, 60, 65, 94n58

LaVergne, TN USA
18 March 2011
220742LV00001B/75/P